PREPARING FOR SURGERY

A MIND-BODY APPROACH TO ENHANCE HEALING AND RECOVERY

D0932039

William W. DEARDORFF, Ph.D.
John L. REEVES II, Ph.D.

New Harbinger Publications, Inc.

Grateful acknowledgment is made to the following for permission to reprint material.

Hospital Stress Rating Scale. Reprinted from *Journal of Human Stress*, June 1977, B.J. Volicer, M.A. Isenberg and M.W. Burns, "Medical-Surgical Differences in Hospital Stress Factors," p. 7, copyright 1977, by permission of Heldref Publications, Washington, DC.

Novaco Anger Inventory-Abbreviated. Reprinted from R. Novaco, *Anger Control: The Development and Evaluation of an Experimental Treatment*, Lexington, MA: D.C. Heath, copyright 1975, by permission of Raymond Novaco, Ph.D.

Trust in Physician Scale. Reprinted from *Psychological Reports*, Volume 67, L.A. Anderson and R.F. Dedrick, "Development of the Trust in Physician Scale: A Measure to Assess Interpersonal Trust in Patient-Physician Relationships," p. 1091-1100, copyright 1990, by permission of L.A. Anderson and R.F. Dedrick.

Ways of Coping Scale. Reprinted from *Social Science and Medicine*, Volume 18, B.J. Felton, T.A. Revenson, and G.A. Hinrichsen, "Stress and Coping in the Explanation of Psychological Adjustment Among Chronically Ill Adults," p. 892-893, copyright 1984, by permission of Elsevier Science, Ltd., The Boulevard, Langford Lane, Kidlington OX5 1GB, UK.

Publisher's Note

This publication is designed to provide accurate and authoritative information in regard to the subject matter covered. It is sold with the understanding that the publisher is not engaged in rendering psychological, financial, legal, or other professional services. If expert assistance or counseling is needed, the services of a competent professional should be sought.

Distributed in the U.S.A. by Publishers Group West; in Canada by Raincoast Books; in Great Britain by Airlift Book Company, Ltd.; in South Africa by Real Books, Ltd.; in Australia by Boobook; and in New Zealand by Tandem Press.

Copyright © 1997 by William W. Deardorff, Ph.D and John L. Reeves II, Ph.D.
New Harbinger Publications, Inc.
5674 Shattuck Avenue
Oakland, CA 94609

Cover design by Blue Design, San Francisco
Text Design by Michele Waters

Library of Congress Catalog Card Number: 96-71159
ISBN 1-57224-071-7 Paperback

Printed in the United States of America on recycled paper.

New Harbinger Publications' Web site address: www.newharbinger.com

10   9   8   7   6   5   4   3   2   1

"In this book, Doctors Deardorff and Reeves have achieved a major communication breakthrough between the patient and the surgeon. I consider this publication essential reading for patients to help themselves, and a key communication and ethical tool for the physician. This is a win-win book!"

>—Robert G. Addison, M.D., Professor, Orthopedic Surgery and Rehabilitation Medicine, Northwestern University Medical School; Past President, American Academy of Pain Medicine; Past President, American Pain Society

"This book ought to be a requirement of hospitals and clinics wherein surgery occurs. Even more importantly, it should be on every surgeon's shelf with prominent reminders to ensure their surgery-candidate patients know about it and are strongly urged to make use of it."

>—Wilbert E. Fordyce, Ph.D., Past President, American Pain Society; Founder and Honorary Member, International Association for the Study of Pain; Co-founder, University of Washington Multidisciplinary Pain Center Treatment Program

"This book is a superb contribution to the self-care literature. Its many strengths include self-assessments to determine one's own coping techniques and concerns about surgery, the many practical coping techniques it contains, and its in-depth explanation of events surrounding surgery. Instead of flowers, send this book to someone you love who is scheduled for surgery!"

>—Betty Ferrell, Ph.D., F.A.A.N., Associate Research Scientist and Chairperson, Southern California Cancer Pain Initiative

"A surgery is more than just operating on a collection of bones and tissue. It is the treatment of a human being at the most serious level. This book addresses the physical and mental aspects of preparing for and recovering from surgery. I wholeheartedly recommend it to anyone facing surgery."

>—Theodore Goldstein, M.D., FACS, Fellow, American Academy of Surgeons; Chief, Department of Orthopedic Surgery, Cedars-Sinai Medical Center, Los Angeles

"Doctors Deardorff and Reeves provide an excellent workbook which should be used by any patient scheduled for surgery."

>—Richard A. Sternbach, Ph.D., Past President, American Pain Society; Honorary Member, International Association for the Study of Pain; author of *Mastering Pain*

To my wife, Janine, for her enduring love, patience, and support. To my sons, James and Paul, for their delightful curiosity and playfulness. To Rachel. To Dr. and Mrs. Jere C. Butterworth, Dr. and Mrs. William T. Deardorff, and Mr. and Mrs. Thomas C. Bedrosian for being great role models.

—William W. Deardorff

To my mom, Ella E. Reeves, whose unconditional love has been the best preparation. To my patients whose courage has pointed the way.

—John L. Reeves II

Acknowledgments

The authors are deeply grateful to those who gave wise and needed guidance in improving the manuscript. We are especially indebted to our editors at New Harbinger, Kayla Sussell, the developmental editor, and Jerry Landis, the copy editor, for transforming our manuscript into this clear and user-friendly book. It is also a pleasure working with Lauren Dockett, Kirk Johnson, Gayle Zanca, and Michele Waters at New Harbinger who have done an excellent job at making this book a reality. Also, to Dr. Allan F. Chino, Lynn Asher, Dr. Louis F. Damis and Dr. Nancy E. Addison for their thoughtful and constructive comments which helped ensure we did not neglect to include any important issues related to preparation for surgery. We would like to give special acknowledgment to our families and colleagues who encouraged us throughout the time we were focused on writing this book. We are deeply grateful for your unselfish support.

Special acknowledgment is given to my mentors Drs. Wilbert Fordyce, Judith Turner, Joan Romano, Saul Spiro, and Cynthia Belar for introducing me to the complex and challenging field of clinical health psychology.

—W.W.D

I want to especially thank Drs. Nancy E. Addison, John C. Liebeskind, Robert G. Addison, Alex B. Caldwell, and Steven B. Graff-Radford for their thoughtful and loving support.

—J.L.R.

Table of Contents

Introduction

Over the past thirty years, scientists and doctors at major university medical centers and hospitals have investigated and explored mind-body techniques to help patients prepare for surgery and more rapid recovery. Until now, these valuable techniques were not readily available to the general public, but only through participation in a research project or specialized program at one of these university hospitals. The preparation for surgery program described in this book was derived from our clinical experience and the scientific literature.

We have summarized the results of over 200 research studies including thousands of patients (Devine 1992; Prokop, Bradley, Burish, Anderson, and Fox 1991; Johnston and Vogele 1993). In addition, we have combined elements of our own experience of working with hundreds of patients facing surgery.

Our program assumes certain things about your surgery that have already been determined and are purposely not covered in this workbook. For example, we assume that you have decided that the surgery is necessary and that you will be scheduled for surgery at a future date. We assume that you have chosen a qualified board-certified surgeon and accredited hospital and that you are comfortable with your choices. We purposely do not cover the topic of living wills and "advanced directives," that is, what you want done in a medical emergency or other medical situation in which you are not capable of responding yourself. These very important issues are covered superbly elsewhere and are listed and annotated for you in the References and Resources section for the Introduction. We direct you specifically to the books by Dr. Bradley; McCabe and Ingersoll; and Inlander and Weiner. Because this workbook is designed to address any type of inpatient or outpatient surgery, presenting details of specific procedures is not possible. Instead we direct you to the excellent books by Drs. Macho and Cable and Dr. Youngson, listed in the References and Resources section, which respectively detail the most common outpatient and inpatient surgeries. In the Appendices and References and Resource sections you will also find a great deal of information pertaining to particular medical conditions and treatments. If you feel that you require more information, contact these organizations.

Our program's goal is to present proven techniques to help you prepare for surgery. We do not discuss detailed theory unless it will help you to understand and develop a specific skill.

Our intention is to give you the ability to design your own preparation for surgery program. You do not need the assistance of a professional to use this book, although some people may find that helpful. The book's usefulness is based on its interactive format and your willingness to practice the techniques and exercises presented. Our program requires you to gather information about yourself and your situation by filling out and analyzing the questionnaires contained in the book. The critical element for obtaining the greatest benefit from this program is to set aside time for regular practice of the mind-body techniques that are presented.

How to Use This Book

Part I, Knowledge is Power: Gathering Information, explains how to design your own mind-body preparation for surgery program. This begins with completing a series of self-assessment questionnaires in Chapter 2. These questionnaires assess such matters as presurgical levels of depression, anxiety, and anger as well as how you feel about the hospital environment and how you cope with stressful situations. The information you obtain from analyzing your answers to these questionnaires is essential for using the techniques in the remainder of the book. This information will help you to create a program individually tailored to your needs, regardless of the type of surgery you are facing.

Chapter 3 helps you to take an active role in gathering information about your surgery. It gives you specific questions and techniques to help you get the information you need. This is essential for designing a successful preparation and recovery program. Due to the stress of dealing with the illness or disease, and the anticipation of surgery, people often neglect to obtain this kind of information, which results in increased uncertainty, worry, and fear.

Part II, Managing the Pain of Surgery, gives you the most up-to-date information on pain control. This is often the area of greatest concern for patients undergoing surgery. You may be worried about adequate pain control before and after the surgery, and whether there is the possibility of becoming addicted to pain medication. Chapter 4 puts you in control of your own pain management.

Part III, Training for Healthy Self-Talk, helps you to prepare your *mind* for surgery by identifying your conscious and unconscious thoughts about your surgery situation. You will learn how to develop the power of healthy thinking and establish coping strategies and affirmations.

Part IV, Mind-Body Techniques, helps you to prepare your *body* for the surgery and the recovery period through the use of the relaxation response, imagery, music, and spiritual awareness. Surgery is a physical stress over which you can exert some control by learning the skills of deep relaxation, imagery, and by listening to special types of music. Chapter 10 explores how spirituality and faith can enhance your surgical recovery. Research shows that all of these techniques can have a very positive impact on your recovery from surgery.

Part V, Taking Control of Your Environment, focuses on time management and effective communication. Chapter 11 teaches you how to manage your time and set healthy priorities. Chapter 12 presents easy-to-learn techniques for communicating with your doctor and other health care professionals as well as techniques on how to be assertive without being aggressive. These skills are very useful when you are interacting with the often bewildering world of medical care.

The Master Task List

The Master Task List that follows this Introduction will help you to successfully complete all aspects of the preparation program appropriate to your needs. As you complete each section of this book, record the date on the Master Task List. This will show you exactly how you are progressing in the program relative to your surgery date. The following principles should be kept in mind.

You will get out of the program what you put into it. Unlike most medical procedures in which you are a passive recipient, the preparation for surgery program requires your active participation. You will benefit from the program to the degree that you are willing to put time into doing the exercises.

You may not need all the material in this book. This program is designed to be used with virtually any type of surgery or stressful medical/dental procedure. It's important that you read *all* of the material, then determine which program components are necessary for you to complete. For instance, many types of breathing exercises are presented in Chapter 7, but most people will use only the one or two exercises that work best for them.

You will need to adjust the speed of your preparation program. Depending on when your surgery is scheduled and when you start the preparation program, you will have to fine-tune how quickly you proceed through the exercises. Most surgeries are scheduled well in advance, so that the timing is flexible. In some cases, however, surgery is recommended as soon as possible. If necessary, much of the information can be gathered quickly. Also, *any* practice of the cognitive and relaxation techniques will be helpful, even if there is not enough time to master these skills completely. Once you are aware of the principles, some of the exercises may also be practiced after the surgery.

Master Task List

Tasks   *Date Completed*

Read Chapter 1   _____

Read Chapter 2   _____

    Complete Questionnaires

        Depression   _____

        Anxiety   _____

        Anger   _____

        Hospital Stress Rating Scale   _____

        Ways of Coping Scale   _____

        Summary Sheet   _____

Read Chapter 3   _____

    Complete Questionnaires

        Surgical Decision Making   _____

        Details of Your Surgery   _____

        Blood Transfusions   _____

        What to Do Before the Surgery   _____

        Questions About the Hospitalization   _____

        Trust-in-Physician Scale   _____

        Making Your Own "Medical Fact Sheet"   _____

        Checklist for the Hospital   _____

Read Chapter 4   _____

    Ask if hospital has pain service   _____

    Talk with your doctor about pain control   _____

Ask your surgeon what to expect   _____

Discuss pain medication options   _____

Review nonmedication approaches   _____

Agree on how to measure your pain   _____

Ask about pain control after discharge   _____

Read Chapter 5   _____

Complete the Self-Talk Journal   _____

Read Chapter 6   _____

Analyze your Self-Talk style   _____

Stop-Challenge-Reframe Self-Talk Journal   _____

Make a list of affirmations   _____

Read Chapter 7   _____

Assess how you breathe   _____

Choose one breathing technique to use   _____

Complete Relaxation Log   _____

Read Chapter 8   _____

Write your imagery script   _____

Prerecord relaxation and imagery   _____

Collect humorous materials   _____

Read Chapter 9   _____

Prepare or purchase audiotape of
anxiety-reducing music   _____

Read Chapter 10   _____

Complete prayer for relaxation   _____

Complete spiritual coping thoughts   _____

Tasks   *Date Completed*

Read Chapter 11   _____

       Complete the Tasks/Reward Sheet   _____

       Complete the Weekly Priority Log   _____

Read Chapter 12   _____

       Review the Personal Bill of Rights   _____

       Record situations for assertiveness   _____

       Record situations for limit-setting   _____

Part I

Knowledge Is Power:
Gathering Information

Part I of this workbook, *Knowledge is Power: Gathering Information*, presents basic information needed to embark upon your mind-body surgical preparation program. The more you know, the more you can do for yourself. Information about surgery enhances recovery from surgery. Chapter 1 explains the rationale and importance of preparing yourself for surgery and using mind-body techniques. Through the use of questionnaires, Chapter 2 helps you to gather information about yourself and your emotional state which will form the basis for your mind-body surgical preparation program. Chapter 3 gives you guidelines for gathering information about your surgery and recovery.

1

Mind-Body Preparation for Surgery: What Is It and Why Do It?

In the United States, approximately fifty million operations are performed each year (Sobel and Ornstein 1996). Of these, 20 percent are in response to an emergency, whereas 80 percent are considered "elective." An elective surgery is one in which the patient and/or the doctor can choose when and where to have the operation. Elective surgeries can range from being "optional" such as removing a wart or cosmetic surgery to "necessary" such as tumor removal, coronary artery bypass, hernia repair, hysterectomy, Caesarean, and some spinal surgeries. Table 1.1 illustrates the most common elective surgeries by category (adapted from Youngson 1993). Our preparation for surgery program is appropriate for any elective surgery done on an inpatient or outpatient basis.

The goal of this book is to provide you with guidelines for coping with your surgery in the healthiest way and, by so doing, increase your chances for the best possible outcome. The following case history illustrates how this works:

> Ted was very nervous about his surgery. His nervousness went beyond
> normal anxiety and he occasionally experienced panic-like attacks. Ted was
> scheduled to have a spinal fusion, a major surgery that includes a lengthy
> postoperative recovery and rehabilitation. He would fluctuate between not
> thinking about the approaching surgery at all to being completely over-
> whelmed even by the idea of it. Because of these fears, he had postponed the
> surgery just days before it was to be done. He felt he had no control over the
> situation; he was afraid of the entire medical environment; and he was at a
> loss as to how to handle his dilemma.

Table 1.1
Common Outpatient and Inpatient Surgeries

Abdominal and Lower Back Surgery
Removal of bladder stones
Removal of bladder tumor
Nephrectomy: removal of a kidney
Kidney transplant
Gastrectomy: removal of part or all of the
  stomach
Appendectomy: removal of the appendix
Colostomy
Splenectomy: removal of the spleen
Liver transplant
Vagotomy: reduction of stomach acid
Hernia repair
Hemorrhoidectomy: removal of hemorrhoids
Cholecystectomy: removal of the gallbladder
Surgery for herniated intervertebral disk
Surgery for aortic aneurysm

Neck Surgery
Radical neck dissection: removal of lymph
  nodes in the neck
Laryngectomy: removal of the larynx
  (voice box)
Thyroidectomy: removal of part of the thyroid
  gland
Tracheostomy
Carotid endarterectomy

Female Reproductive System
Dilatation and curettage
Hysterectomy: removal of the uterus
Induced abortion
Episiotomy
Childbirth by Caesarean section
Surgery for ectopic pregnancy
Female sterilization
Removal of fibroids in the uterus
Surgery for cervical precancer
Drainage of breast abscess or cyst
Radical mastectomy
Lumpectomy

Male Reproductive System
Circumcision: removal of the foreskin of the
  penis
Vasectomy: male sterilization
Prostatectomy: removal of part or all of the
  prostate gland
Orchiectomy: removal of a testis

Cosmetic Surgery
Removal of birthmarks, tattoos, and keloid
  scars
Removal of warts
Rhinoplasty: reshaping the nose
Blepharoplasty: removing bags around
  the eyes
Rhytidectomy: facelift
Hair transplants and implants
Breast reconstruction
Breast enlargement
Breast reduction
Removing excess tissue and fat from the
  abdomen

Surgery to the Head
Removal of a basal cell carcinoma
Surgery to treat otosclerotic deafness
Washing out nasal sinuses
Tonsillectomy: removal of the tonsils
Tooth extraction
Root canal treatment

Heart Surgery
Heart valve replacement
Coronary artery bypass
Pacemaker implantation
Heart-lung transplant

Arm and Leg Surgery
Removal of a bunion
Surgery to treat varicose veins in the leg
Meniscectomy: surgery for knee cartilage
  damage
Surgery for hand contracture
Surgery for carpal tunnel syndrome
Bone fracture treatment
Hip replacement
Leg amputation

Surgery to the Chest
Pneumonectomy: lung removal
Drainage of lung abscess

Surgery Inside the Skull
Removal of a brain tumor or blood clot
Removal of an abscess in the brain
Cataract surgery
Correction of a squint (strabismus)

Ted was referred to us by his surgeon for the preparation for surgery program. In working with Ted, we covered all the skills and exercises outlined in this book. Through the program he got his questions answered, became more assertive about his medical needs, learned how to control stress and pain, changed his thinking about the surgery, and increased his overall sense of control. He began to feel more like a "partner" in his medical treatment than a passive recipient or "victim." At the end of the program he was actually looking forward to "getting beyond" the surgery and beginning his rehabilitation. The surgery was completed successfully and Ted did very well throughout the hospitalization. During his post-operative rehabilitation, he was able to use the skills he had learned to facilitate a smooth recovery.

Why Prepare for Surgery?

When helping people to prepare for surgery, we are often asked, "Why should I bother preparing for surgery?" The following sentiment from one of our patients is representative of many:

"Why do I need to prepare for surgery? I think I know what will happen. I'll go into the hospital, they'll put me to sleep, they'll fix the problem, I'll wake up, and then I'll go home. Who needs to prepare for that?"

Many people, including some surgeons, take a very matter-of-fact view of surgery such as that above. We term this the "auto-mechanic" view, which likens surgery to fixing a car. Given the fact that you are a human being, which is much more than a collection of bone and tissue, this notion of how surgery works could not be further from the truth. The fact is that surgery is stressful and it can have a significant impact on your mind, body, and emotions.

Using mind-body techniques to prepare for surgery, and to cope with the postsurgical recovery period, can have very positive benefits, such as the following:

- Less anxiety both before and after surgery

- Fewer complications related to the surgery and recovery

- Less pain and less need for postoperative pain medication

- Quicker return to health

- Shorter stay in the hospital

Doctors Marie Johnston and Claus Vogele (1993) reviewed almost ninety scientific research studies on psychological preparation for surgery and concluded, "There is now substantial agreement that psychological preparation for surgery is beneficial to patients." In another major review of 191 studies dating from 1963 until the present, Dr. E. C. Devine (1992) concluded that the positive benefits outlined above do, in fact, occur with surgical preparation

What Are Patients' Main Worries About Surgery?

The following are the primary concerns of patients facing surgery:

- Whether the operation will be a success
- How long it will be before there is a return to normal
- Feeling "unwell" after the surgery
- Being away from home
- How one's spouse will cope
- How one's children will cope
- Dying during the operation
- What is physically wrong
- Pain after the operation
- Being unconscious
- Family worrying
- Doctors explaining the procedure
- Waking up during the operation
- Fear that the doctor will make a mistake during the operation

(Based on Johnston 1988.)

programs. These studies provide impressive scientific support for the conclusion that *mind-body preparation for surgery can improve outcome and enhance overall recovery and healing*. Mind-body preparation for surgery and postoperative recovery is especially important given the ongoing national changes in the delivery of health care. As you may know, there is a strong trend today toward shorter hospital stays and more outpatient surgeries.

Outpatient Surgery

In 1997, nearly three-quarters of all Americans with health insurance are enrolled in health maintenance organizations (HMOs). Today, more than half of all surgical procedures in the United States are performed on an outpatient basis (*Los Angeles Times*, 1/20/97, p. A 17). These numbers translate into over two hundred kinds of operations that require no hospital stay (Macho 1994).

It's no secret that this dramatic shift to HMOs away from the traditional American fee-for-service delivery of health care was fueled by skyrocketing health costs. And, clearly, outpatient surgery reduces medical costs. What is not as well known is that the shift to outpatient surgery was caused by several factors—not just the need to contain costs.

Since it is more than likely that your surgery will be done on an outpatient basis, it might interest you to know some of the other causes.

Surgery and High Technology

In the past twenty-five years many operations have become much safer and easier to perform because of high-tech instruments that require less-invasive procedures. For example, many abdominal procedures that formerly could be done only with huge incisions now use tiny video cameras that require only tiny incisions. Orthopedic surgeons explore and operate *inside* joints using special equipment called arthroscopes. Imaging techniques like magnetic resonance imaging (MRI) and computerized tomography (CT) scans allow surgeons to see *inside* the body and to pinpoint troublesome areas with such accuracy that a biopsy can be performed with a thin needle.

Improved Pain Medication and Anesthesia

Once, the use of general anesthesia meant that the patient had to stay in the hospital to be carefully watched for postanesthesia nausea and vomiting. Now, general anesthesia is used for over half of all outpatient surgeries (Macho 1994). The differences are due to the new faster-acting agents that do not cause vomiting. These newer drugs also have shorter recovery times. Also, today, long-acting local anesthetics are directly injected into incision sites.

In addition, new oral pain medications are very effective, safe, and as easily monitored at home as in a hospital.

Increased Patient Control and Less Patient Anxiety

Many people, given the choice, would much rather choose outpatient surgery than inpatient because hospital stays can be so disruptive to work or school. Furthermore, when surgery is performed in a center that does only surgeries, less time is spent waiting for a hospital's operating facilities. Shorter waits mean less preoperative anxiety and tension. Finally, outpatient surgeries consistently report fewer postoperative infections than inpatient surgeries do, probably because patients are not exposed to bacteria normally present in hospital wards (Macho 1994).

Outpatient Responsibilities and Managed Health Care

There is no doubt that having surgery is right up there with changing jobs or getting a divorce as a major life stressor. But if you approach your surgery equipped with all the information you can acquire about what to expect, before, during, and after the operation, you will be in the best possible position to contribute to your own recovery. Managed care programs expect patients to play a more responsible role in their health care than traditional fee-for-service providers. Patients' friends and families are also expected to provide more significant support than previously was the case.

HMO patients are often given checklists of all the presurgical procedures they will need to take care of before their operations. They usually have to spend a certain amount of time having lab tests or X rays. These tests may require numerous visits to various medical offices and a lot of waiting that can be fairly frustrating. Hang in there. Bring a friend or a good book along to make the waiting more tolerable.

Currently, some of the larger HMOs are establishing new programs and procedures specifically set up to deal with patients' presurgical concerns. Other HMOs leave it up to the individual patients themselves to find out what they need to know. Our preparation for surgery program should be useful for both groups.

The questionnaires provided in Chapters 2 and 3 will give you a headstart in taking on responsibility for your own care and recovery. Be prepared to assert yourself in the quest for information. For example, most anesthesiologists are extremely busy people. You may not be able to schedule a presurgical conference with the doctor who will take care of your anesthesia

The Physical Stress of Surgery

Surgery is a major physical stressor. In addition to pain, there are other significant body reactions that occur which may impair healing.

For instance, chemicals released from the tissues injured during surgery can cause a variety of "stress hormone" responses. These stress-hormone responses result in negative occurrences in the body such as the following:

- The breakdown of body tissue
- Increased metabolic rate
- Blood clotting
- Water retention
- Impaired immune function
- The "fight or flight" stress reaction

These stress-hormone responses can be minimized using the mind-body techniques described in this book.

during your surgery. In fact, that doctor may not even be known until the day of your surgery. You will, however, be able to question someone who is an anesthesiologist at the surgery center. You may have to insist on your right to do so, but it will be worth it.

The same principle holds true for all of the questionnaires in this book: they may be troublesome to complete and you may have to talk to people who will not be directly involved in your surgery. Nevertheless, all HMOs should have competent staff available to answer all of your presurgical questionnaires and the resulting gain in your knowledge will be greatly to your advantage and will decrease your presurgical anxieties considerably.

The Stress of Surgery

In recent years the technology of surgery has advanced dramatically while large-scale use of mind-body preparation techniques has lagged behind. The goals of surgery are to save lives, reduce or eliminate pain, and improve the quality of life. Even with such positive goals, surgery causes major stress primarily around two issues: First, there is the significant illness or problem that is the focus of the surgical treatment; and second, a significant invasive medical procedure is being recommended. It is important to acknowledge how stressful these challenges can be and a preparation for surgery program must address both of these issues.

Surgical Stress and Your Mind

Surgical stress can result from how you *think* about the operation and related issues. Several studies have examined the primary worries patients have about surgery. Doctor J. E. Johnson found that patients' main worries rank in the order shown in the sidebar entitled "What Are Patients' Main Worries About Surgery?" (page 12).

In our clinical experience with preparation for surgery programs, these worries are very common but often are not acknowledged. They may occur at a very conscious level, or more unconsciously, and they can be the source of significant emotional distress both before and after surgery. Worries can also be caused by issues beyond the actual surgery itself. Such concerns generally involve the *meaning* of the surgery to the patient. The following case history illustrates this point:

Connie thought she was prepared for her hysterectomy and she was trying to keep an optimistic attitude. Even so, she was experiencing periodic crying spells for no apparent reason and not feeling "quite right"—i.e., low energy, sleep problems, weight loss, wanting to be alone, and decreased sex drive. She came to our program at the urging of a friend who had found it useful. During the course of the program, it became clear that she was suffering from depression without being fully aware of it. For Connie, the prospect of the hysterectomy carried significant negative weight in terms of her fears about a change in her body image and the procedure's possible impact on her sexual functioning. These fears and their concomitant emotional reactions are often aroused by the prospect of this operation.

Unlike Ted's case, Connie's stress and depression were related not to the surgery itself, but rather to the *meaning* she attached to the operation. Thus, the preparation for surgery program focused on relieving her depression. This was done by giving her accurate information about the surgery and dispelling some myths about how her life would be after the hysterectomy.

Cognitive (thought-related) preparation for surgery will help you to identify the conscious and unconscious worries you may have about the operation and your recovery. Cognitive strategies include such techniques as identifying healthy and unhealthy thoughts, thought stopping, thought substitution and rehearsal, affirmations, and coping skills

Does Psychological Stress Hamper Healing?

According to new research there is now direct evidence that psychological stress has a negative impact on healing. Scientists have known for some time that stress can prevent our immune systems from working at optimal levels thereby making us more vulnerable to infection. Now it appears that stress actually can slow the healing of wounds. Of course, this is an important finding for anyone undergoing surgery.

For instance, Drs. Linn, Klimas, and Linn (1988) found that people who experienced more everyday life stress had more difficult recoveries from surgery. Also, Dr. Kiecolts-Glaser (1995) and colleagues studied a group of healthy women who had been caring for a disabled husband or parent an average of seven hours per day for seven years. This "high stress" group was compared with a similar group of women without similar stress. All of the women in the study underwent the removal of a small piece of skin from the inner arm below the elbow. The study found that the wounds of the women in the high-stress group took about nine days longer to heal than the other group! There were no other factors found that could explain these results except for the difference in stress levels.

If stress can slow down the healing time of these small wounds, you can imagine what impact it might have on the healing time after major surgery.

development. These techniques, once mastered, will help you to manage effectively the mental stress of surgery and recovery.

Surgical Stress and Your Body

However positive its goal, surgery can temporarily cause serious physical stress. It generally causes significant trauma to the tissues which makes the body's healing process more difficult. In addition, while the body is trying to heal, it must also continue to fight off infection as well as manage pain.

The stress of surgery on the body can also cause physical reactions not directly related to the procedure. One such reaction is the "physical stress response." Stress responses occur when we feel threatened. In the case of surgery, this reaction can take place both before and after the operation. Physical stress reactions occur in varying intensities, and the person experiencing them may or may not be aware of them.

The stress response is also termed the "fight or flight response" because it is the set of physical reactions that occurs when one is threatened by something believed to be dangerous. For instance, think of how you would feel if you were hiking in the woods and you suddenly came across a large snake on the trail. You would immediately experience the "fight or flight" physical reaction. This includes such physical events as "cardiovascular reactivity" (an increase in heart rate and blood pressure), the release of stress hormones into the blood stream, rapid breathing, sweating palms, and tense muscles. This set of physical reactions is a primitive response necessary for survival in threatening situations; that is, when you have the choice of fighting or running away to save yourself. But this same set of reactions can occur whether or not the situation actually presents a real danger. We need only *believe* that there might be danger to experience the "fight or flight" response.

All of us have experienced different levels of the physical stress response. One common example occurs when you are stuck in traffic knowing that you are very late for an important appointment. Or, consider how you feel when you are scheduled to take a difficult test or give a speech in front of a large audience, especially if you are not prepared. These are the kinds of situations that activate the physiological events described above due to anticipating a threatening situation. Maintaining such a stress response for an extended period of time can be detrimental to your physical health as well as facilitating depression and anxiety.

This preparation for surgery program teaches you how to control the physical stress response both before and after the surgery by using such techniques as deep relaxation through breathing exercises, visualization, distraction, and selective attention. These techniques can improve the entire surgical process and postoperative recovery.

Surgical Stress and Your Emotions

It is very common to experience a number of emotional reactions both before and after an invasive medical procedure. These emotions are generally related to various worries that you might have about the surgery as well as the illness or disease for which the surgery is indicated. In our experience, the most common emotions and their causes are as follows:

Anxiety

- Uncertainty about the future
- Expectations about functioning after the surgery
- Being in a strange place
- Being in embarrassing situations (e.g., nudity and toileting)
- Not being in control
- Being away from home
- Worry about family members
- Not understanding issues about the surgery

Depression

- Related to the illness that requires the surgery
- Related to feeling helpless about the surgery
- Related to financial or personal stressors
- Related to inability to work

Fear

- Of medical procedures
- Of doctors and health professionals
- Of pain and discomfort
- Of being in the strange hospital setting
- Of coming home after the operation to recover
- Of dying

Anger

- About your need for surgery

Are You an Information Seeker or Information Avoider?

Do you tend to agree or disagree with the following statements?

1. Investigating books, magazines, and television programs about my medical problems and surgeries makes me feel more confident and in control.
2. I tend to gather very specific and detailed information about my health-related issues.
3. Detailed medical information does not bother me.

Generally research has shown that patients who possess accurate information about their impending surgery do better overall. Realistic information allows patients to develop accurate expectations and effective coping strategies.

Further investigations have demonstrated that some people do better with very specific and detailed information about their surgery (information-seekers) while others do better with very general information (information-avoiders). This depends on your coping style.

Review your answers to the statements above. If you tended to agree with the statements, then you are more of an information-seeker. If you tended to disagree with the statements, then you are more of an information-avoider. This workbook is adaptable to your unique coping style. Simply gather the amount and detail of information that feels comfortable for you.

- At your doctors, nurses, or the hospital setting

- At your family members for "not understanding"

- At your body for "failing you"

Emotional reactions are major factors that can affect your ability to cope before and after the surgery, your pain threshold, your complications after the surgery, and your recovery from surgery.

To prepare emotionally for surgery you must identify the worries *behind* the emotions and address them. The preparation for surgery program will help you to manage your emotional responses in a nonthreatening and healthy manner.

Surgical Stress and Your Environment

Going through a surgery can have a significant impact on the many environments in which you live including your home and workplace. Your family, friends, and colleagues at work can all be affected by your surgery. Other important environments associated with surgery include the hospital setting and your insurance company.

In our experience, a person facing surgery may seldom think about these "environmental" issues even though these can cause significant stress if not addressed.

Environmental stress might include such matters as:

- How you and your family will react to your time in the hospital and your recovery period at home

- Whether your friends will try to offer too much or too little support during your surgery and recovery

- Whether you will need special rehabilitation treatment after the surgery

- How you will respond to the hospital setting

- How you will work with your doctor's office

- How your employer and work colleagues will respond to your time away and your ultimate return to work

- How secure your job and your financial situation are

- Will your insurance company provide for part or full coverage for treatments related to the surgery and recovery

The preparation for surgery program helps you to prepare your environments for your surgeries by addressing these issues. The goal of preparing these environments is to decrease ambiguity and increase one's personal sense of control to reduce stress and enhance healing.

2

Assessing Yourself Mentally, Emotionally, and Physically Prior to Surgery

Different people need to prepare for surgery in different ways. This book helps you to design and complete your own, individualized preparation for surgery program to accomplish the positive outcome you hope to achieve.

The first task is to gather and evaluate information about yourself to help you design your program. How you prepare for surgery will depend on such things as:

- What kind of person you are and how you generally handle stress

- What type of condition or illness you are having surgery for

- How long you have been suffering from the illness or condition

- How the condition or illness has affected your life in terms of work, family relationships, and recreational activities

- How extensive the surgery is and how long the recovery period may be

- What experiences you have had in the past with surgery, medical treatment, and hospitalization

This chapter and the next assess important information about you and your surgery. Complete each section fully. The information will be used throughout the preparation program. Also, you may refer to some of the questionnaires again to determine the progress of your preparation.

What Is Clinical Depression?

Clinical depression differs from normal "sadness" and involves symptoms such as those listed below. It is often treated with psychotherapy and antidepressant medications. Treatment of depression prior to surgery can be crucial. Common symptoms of clinical depression include:

- A mood which is depressed, sad, hopeless, or irritable and may include periodic crying spells

- Poor appetite or significant weight loss or increased appetite or significant weight gain

- Too much or too little sleep

- Feeling agitated (restless) or sluggish (low energy or fatigue)

- Loss of interest or pleasure in usual activities; social isolation

- Decreased sex drive

- Feelings of worthlessness and/or guilt

- Problems with concentration or memory

- Thoughts of death or suicide, or wishing to die

Depression

Our experience and many studies suggest that depression has a negative impact on your surgery and recovery. Clinical depression goes beyond normal sadness or feeling "down" for a few days. It includes symptoms such as those listed in this sidebar entitled "What Is Clinical Depression?"

Depression ranges from sadness to clinical depression. It is beyond the scope and purpose of this book to discuss the many reasons for depression. Generally, it accompanies a feeling of having little or no control over one's environment or situation. This can result from dealing with an ongoing illness, family or job stress, or the stress of undergoing medical treatments. As can be seen in the following case example, clinical depression should be treated prior to surgery, if possible. The questionnaire following the case example will help you determine your level of depression.

Brenda was scheduled to undergo elective cosmetic surgery. Since she was somewhat apprehensive about the surgery, her doctor suggested that she complete a brief preparation for surgery program. It was apparent from her initial interview and analysis of the depression questionnaire that she was clinically depressed. She had undergone a series of stressors recently and had been treated for depression in the remote past with antidepressant medicines. In trying to manage her current stress, she had ignored her worsening symptoms of depression.

After talking with Brenda, it was decided that she would postpone her surgery until the depression could be treated properly. Since the surgery was entirely elective, the timing of it was under her control. Her depression was successfully treated with a combination of antidepressant medicine and short-term counseling. She then completed the preparation for surgery program and scheduled the surgery. Her surgery and recovery went well and she considered it a complete success.

The Depression Questionnaire

Using the following scale for each of the listed symptoms, circle the number that best indicates how much you have experienced this type of feeling over the past one to two weeks. Make sure you answer all the questions. If you feel unsure about any, indicate your best guess.

0 = Not at all   1 = Somewhat   2 = Moderately   3 = A lot

1. Do you feel sad, low, blue, or unhappy?	0	1	2	3
2. Do you feel hopeless or discouraged about the future?	0	1	2	3
3. Do you feel useless or believe yourself to be a failure?	0	1	2	3
4. Do you feel inadequate or inferior to others?	0	1	2	3
5. Do you feel guilty or blame yourself for everything?	0	1	2	3
6. Do you find it difficult to make decisions?	0	1	2	3
7. Do you feel frustrated and irritable?	0	1	2	3
8. Have you lost interest in other people or your usual activities?	0	1	2	3
9. Do you feel unmotivated and find it difficult to do things?	0	1	2	3
10. Do you think you're looking old, unattractive, or ugly?	0	1	2	3
11. Have you lost your appetite or had a change in weight not due to dieting?	0	1	2	3
12. Do you have trouble falling asleep, or do you wake up during the night, earlier than you would like?	0	1	2	3
13. Do you feel tired much of the time?	0	1	2	3
14. Have you had crying spells or felt like crying but couldn't?	0	1	2	3
15. Have you lost your interest in sex?	0	1	2	3
16. Do you worry often about your general health even beyond the upcoming surgery?	0	1	2	3

17. Do you have thoughts about killing your-
    self or do you think you might be better
    off dead?   0   1   2   3

Add up your total score for the 17 symptoms and record it here: _____

The total score will be somewhere between 0 (answering "Not at all" to each item) and 51 (answering "A lot" for each item). Use the following key to interpret your score:

Total Score	*Degree of Depression*
0–4	Minimal or no depression
6–11	Borderline depression
12–21	Mild depression
22–31	Moderate depression
32–51	Severe depression

If you have had thoughts about killing yourself or scored in the "severe" range of depression, you should consult a qualified mental health professional.

If your depression score is in the moderate to severe range, you may want to discuss the possibility of postponing your surgery until the depression can be treated. Treatment for depression is often appropriate as part of the preparation for surgery program. The goal of treatment is to give you a sense of control over stressful situations and to alleviate as many of the above symptoms as possible. Presurgical depression can be associated with continued or more severe depression after surgery, and can negatively influence your ability to recover from the surgery.

Treatment will depend on the severity of the depression. For moderate to severe depression, treatment with antidepressant medications is often appropriate. These medications work best when used in conjunction with "cognitive" techniques (changing thoughts). For milder depression, medication is usually not necessary and the depression may respond well to cognitive techniques alone. These cognitive techniques are discussed in Chapter 6.

Anxiety

Anxiety is probably the most thoroughly researched emotion with regard to preparation for surgery and surgical outcomes. As stated by Dr. David Horne, "Patients' anxious reactions to an invasive surgical procedure are major factors affecting pre- and postoperative adjustment." (Horne 1994). Numerous studies have demonstrated elevated anxiety and stress ratings for presurgical patients. It has also been found that for many patients anxiety scores after surgery may continue to be high. When the anxiety or stress response is significant and maintained for a long period of time (pre- and postsurgically), it is not only distressing for the patient, it also can have a negative impact on the speed and quality of surgical wound healing.

Anxiety can range from nervousness to full panic attacks. It is normal to experience some anticipatory anxiety before surgery as with any other stressful event (e.g., test or examination, public speaking, physical threat). The following self-assessment questionnaire will help you to determine your level of anxiety:

The Anxiety Questionnaire

The following is a list of symptoms people sometimes have in conjunction with surgery. For each of the symptoms, circle the number that best indicates how much you have been bothered by this type of feeling during the past week.

0 = Not at all   1 = Somewhat   2 = Moderately   3 = A lot

Anxious Thoughts and Feelings

1. Anxiety, nervousness, worry, fear, or apprehension	0	1	2	3
2. Feeling that things around you are strange or unreal	0	1	2	3
3. Feeling detached from all or part of your body	0	1	2	3
4. Sudden unexpected panic episodes	0	1	2	3
5. A sense that something bad is about to happen or of impending doom	0	1	2	3
6. Feeling tense, stressed, or "uptight"	0	1	2	3
7. Difficulty concentrating	0	1	2	3
8. Racing thoughts; your mind jumps from one thing to the next	0	1	2	3
9. Frightening thoughts, or fantasies	0	1	2	3
10. Feeling that you're about to lose control	0	1	2	3
11. Fear of going crazy	0	1	2	3
12. Fear of fainting or passing out	0	1	2	3
13. Fear of being alone or abandoned	0	1	2	3
14. Fear of criticism or disapproval	0	1	2	3

Physical Symptoms

15.	Skipping, racing, or pounding of the heart	0	1	2	3
16.	Pain, pressure, or tightness in the chest	0	1	2	3
17.	Tingling or numbness in the toes, fingers, or around the mouth	0	1	2	3
18.	Butterflies, upset, or discomfort in the stomach	0	1	2	3
19.	Constipation or diarrhea	0	1	2	3
20.	Restlessness or jumpiness	0	1	2	3
21.	Tight, tense muscles	0	1	2	3
22.	Sweating not brought on by heat	0	1	2	3
23.	A lump in the throat	0	1	2	3
24.	Trembling or shaking	0	1	2	3
25.	Rubbery or "jelly" legs	0	1	2	3
26.	Feeling dizzy, light-headed, or off balance	0	1	2	3
27.	Shallow breathing or "gulping" air when you breathe	0	1	2	3
28.	Cold and clammy hands	0	1	2	3
29.	Hot or cold spells	0	1	2	3
30.	Feeling tired or easily exhausted	0	1	2	3
31.	Trembling voice when you speak	0	1	2	3

Add up your total score for the 31 symptoms: _____

After you have completed the anxiety questionnaire, add up your total score for all of the symptoms. Your score will range somewhere from 0 (answering "Not at all" to all of the questions) to 93 (if you answered "A lot" to all symptoms). The following key will help determine your level of anxiety.

Total Score	Degree of Anxiety
0–4	Minimal or no anxiety
6–11	Borderline anxiety
12–21	Mild anxiety
22–31	Moderate anxiety
32–51	Severe anxiety
52–93	Extreme anxiety or panic

The results of the anxiety questionnaire are also useful to determine how your anxiety expresses itself. In the Anxiety Questionnaire there are two categories of symptoms—Anxious Thoughts and Feelings, and Physical Symptoms. Scan your scores to determine in which category you express more anxiety. This can help you to understand how your anxiety affects you and what kind of work you need to do to reduce it through the preparation program. For example, the results of the Anxiety Questionnaire helped us plan a preparation for surgery program in the following case:

John required prostate surgery and was suffering from severe anxiety about the operation. His anxiety included such symptoms as constant worry, episodes of hyperventilation, and the feeling that he was going to "pass out." On his Anxiety Questionnaire, his score in the Anxious Thoughts and Feelings section was moderate to high, and in the very high range in the Physical Symptoms section. During the course of the program, it became evident that his anxiety/hyperventilation episodes had a predictable cycle. First he would unconsciously, and then consciously, begin to think about catastrophic "what ifs" related to the

What Is Clinical Anxiety?

Clinical anxiety differs from common nervousness or stress. It is an excessive, pervasive anxiety characterized by persistent worry, restlessness, fatigue, irritability, muscle tension, sleep disturbances, and loss of concentration. Clinical anxiety significantly impairs interaction in social, occupational, and other areas. It is far more severe than the normal anticipatory anxiety surrounding surgery.

Panic attacks are a form of extreme anxiety. Among the symptoms of a panic attack are hyperventilation, shortness of breath, a sense of impending doom, dizziness, and feeling faint. Panic attacks do not usually result from a specific fear and often occur spontaneously.

Severe anxiety is most effectively treated with psychological methods such as relaxation training and changing thoughts, and, occasionally, with medication. It should be addressed in the preparation for surgery program.

surgery. As these thoughts progressed, his breathing would become more and more shallow and rapid. This would cause increasingly severe physical symptoms. The preparation program gave John the skills to stop and change the worrisome thoughts, and to relax and stop the hyperventilation and associated symptoms. Although the hospitalization and recovery periods were difficult for him, he was able to get through them without experiencing a single episode of hyperventilation.

For more precise data, you can determine your average score for each category. To get the average for anxious thoughts and feelings add the total of all responses and divide the number by 14. For physical symptoms divide the total by 17 to obtain the average. Compare the two average scores to see whether you express anxiety more physically or mentally.

Anger

Although there is little current research, our experience suggests that anger can have a significant impact on your surgical experience. Some anger or irritation is normal if you have a chronic illness which affects many aspects of your life. This anger may be difficult to express because there is no specific "thing" at which to be angry. Therefore, it is often expressed towards yourself and those around you. You may find yourself angry at family, friends, doctors, nurses, hospital personnel, and others. Expressing your anger in an unhealthy way can cause conflicts before and after your surgery.

Barbara's anger was getting in the way of her medical treatment. She was scheduled to undergo blood vessel surgery that would require several days in the hospital for postoperative rehabilitation. She had a "short fuse" and had many explosive interactions with her doctors and their office personnel. After a while, she noticed that people tried to avoid her when she called the doctor's office or scheduled a visit. This made her even angrier and more aggressive. In her preparation for surgery program, we emphasized anger management and effective communication skills (assertive versus aggressive). We pointed out to her that people were backing away from her to avoid her angry outbursts, and that this made her increasingly dissatisfied with her treatment. Moreover, she was actually receiving less attentive medical care as a result. The communication skills training and relaxation exercises enabled her to control her anger and improve her interactions with the medical staff, which resulted in better treatment for her throughout her surgical experience.

Dr. Raymond Novaco (1975) has developed the Novaco Anger Inventory which will help you to assess the degree of anger you may be experiencing. Awareness of your level of anger and irritability will help you to reduce unnecessary distress as you prepare for your surgery. (Refer to Chapters 5, 6, 7, and 12 for information on these issues).

Novaco Anger Inventory*

Instructions. Read the following twenty-five potentially upsetting situations. For each situation, estimate the level of anger you would feel using the following scale:

0 = You would feel little or no annoyance   3 = You would feel quite angry

1 = You would feel a little irritated   4 = You would feel very angry

2 = You would feel moderately upset

As you describe how you would react to each of the following situations, make your best guess about the level of irritation/anger you would experience even though details are omitted.

1. You unpack an appliance you have just bought, plug it in, and discover it doesn't work   0   1   2   3   4

2. Being overcharged by a repairman who has you over a barrel   0   1   2   3   4

3. Being singled out for correction, when the actions of others go unnoticed   0   1   2   3   4

4. Getting your car stuck in the mud or snow   0   1   2   3   4

5. You are talking to someone and they don't answer you   0   1   2   3   4

6. Someone pretends to be something they are not   0   1   2   3   4

7. While you are struggling to carry four cups of coffee to your table at a cafeteria, someone bumps into you, spilling the coffee   0   1   2   3   4

8. You have hung up your clothes, but someone knocks them to the floor and fails to pick them up   0   1   2   3   4

9. You are hounded by a salesperson from the moment you walk into a store   0   1   2   3   4

10. You have made arrangements to go somewhere with a person who backs off at the last minute and leaves you hanging   0   1   2   3   4

11. Being joked or teased about   0   1   2   3   4

12. Your car is stalled at a traffic light, and the guy behind you keeps blowing his horn   0   1   2   3   4

13. You accidentally make the wrong kind of turn in a parking lot. As you get out of your car someone yells at you, "Where did you learn to drive?"   0   1   2   3   4

14. Someone makes a mistake and blames it on you   0   1   2   3   4

15. You are trying to concentrate, but a person near you is tapping his or her foot   0   1   2   3   4

16. You lend someone an important book or tool, and he or she fails to return it   0   1   2   3   4

17. You have had a busy day, and the person you live with starts to complain about how you forgot to do something that you agreed to do   0   1   2   3   4

18. You are trying to discuss something important with your mate or partner who isn't giving you a chance to express your feelings   0   1   2   3   4

19. You are in a discussion with someone who persists in arguing about a topic they know very little about   0   1   2   3   4

20. Someone sticks his nose into an argument between you and someone else   0   1   2   3   4

21. You need to get somewhere quickly, but the car in front of you is going 25 mph in a 40 mph zone, and you can't pass   0   1   2   3   4

22. Stepping on a gob of chewing gum   0   1   2   3   4

23. Being mocked by a small group of people as you pass them   0   1   2   3   4

24. In a hurry to get somewhere, you tear a good pair of slacks on a sharp object   0   1   2   3   4

25. You use your last dime to make a phone call, but you are disconnected before you finish dialing and the dime is lost   0   1   2   3   4

Add your scores on all items to get your total score: _____

Your total score will fall somewhere between 0 (answering "No annoyance" to all of the items) to 100 (answering "Very angry" to all of the items). Use the following key to interpret your total anger score.

Total Score	*Degree of Anger*
0–45	**Very Low Anger.** You have a very low level of anger and annoyance. Are you sure you are that relaxed?
46–55	**Low Anger.** You are more peaceful than the average person.
56–75	**Average Anger. You experience an average amount of anger in response to annoyances.**
76–85	**Substantial Anger.** You frequently react with anger at a level far above the average person.
86–100	**Intense Anger.** You are plagued by frequent intense furious reactions that do not quickly disappear. Your anger may often get out of control.

* Novaco Anger Inventory-Abbreviated. Reprinted from Novaco, R. 1975. *Anger Control: The Development and Evaluation of an Experimental Treatment*, Lexington, MA: D.C. Heath, Used by permission of Raymond Novaco, Ph.D.

Hospital Stress

Going to the hospital, either as an inpatient or outpatient, can be stressful in different ways to different people. Dr. Beverly Volicer (1977) investigated the types of events related to hospitalization that surgical patients have found to be stressful. She categorized these stressors as:

- Unfamiliarity of surroundings
- Loss of independence
- Separation from spouse or significant other
- Financial problems
- Isolation from other people
- Lack of information
- Threat of severe illness
- Separation from family
- Problems with medications

To become aware of those aspects of the entire process that might be stressful for you is an important step in preparing for surgery and hospitalization. The Hospital Stress Rating Scale (HSRS) was originally developed by Dr. Volicer to evaluate the stress associated with various aspects of hospitalization. In Dr. Volicer's research, the HSRS was completed by patients after they had been admitted to the hospital. For the purposes of preparing for surgery we have patients complete the HSRS before hospitalization.

Please complete and score the following HSRS to determine your areas of stress associated with hospitalization:

Hospital Stress Rating Scale*

Instructions. Think about each hospitalization-related event below and decide if it would be stressful for you. If it would be stressful for you, or has been in the past, check the line next to it. The "Mean Value" column will be completed later.

	Check here if stressful	*Mean Value*
Unfamiliarity of Surroundings		
1. Having strangers sleep in the same room with you	_____	_____
2. Having to sleep in a strange bed	_____	_____
3. Having strange machines around	_____	_____
4. Being awakened in the night by the nurse	_____	_____
5. Being aware of unusual smells around you	_____	_____
6. Being in a room that is too cold or too hot	_____	_____
7. Having to eat cold or tasteless food	_____	_____
8. Being cared for by an unfamiliar doctor	_____	_____
Loss of Independence		
9. Having to eat at different times than you usually do	_____	_____
10. Having to wear a hospital gown	_____	_____
11. Having to be assisted with bathing	_____	_____
12. Not being able to get newspapers, radio, or TV when you want them	_____	_____
13. Having a roommate who has too many visitors	_____	_____
14. Having to stay in bed or the same room all day	_____	_____
15. Having to be assisted with a bedpan	_____	_____
16. Not having your call light answered	_____	_____
17. Being fed through tubes	_____	_____
18. Thinking you may lose your sight	_____	_____

Separation from Spouse or Significant Other

19. Worrying about your spouse being away from you   _____   _____

20. Missing your spouse   _____   _____

Financial Problems

21. Thinking about losing income because of your illness   _____   _____

22. Not having enough insurance to pay for your hospitalization   _____   _____

Isolation from Other People

23. Having a roommate who is seriously ill or cannot talk with you   _____   _____

24. Having a roommate who is unfriendly   _____   _____

25. Not having friends visit you   _____   _____

26. Not being able to call family or friends on the phone   _____   _____

27. Having the staff be in too much of a hurry   _____   _____

28. Thinking you might lose your hearing   _____   _____

Lack of Information

29. Thinking you might have pain because of surgery or test procedures   _____   _____

30. Not knowing when to expect things will be done to you   _____   _____

31. Having nurses or doctors talk too fast or use words you can't understand   _____   _____

32. Not having your questions answered by staff   _____   _____

33. Not knowing the results or reasons for your treatments   _____   _____

34. Not knowing for sure what illnesses you have   _____   _____

35. Not being told what your diagnosis is   _____   _____

	Check here if stressful	*Mean Value*

Threat of Severe Illness

36. Thinking your appearance might be changed after your hospitalization   _____   _____

37. Being put in the hospital because of an accident   _____   _____

38. Knowing you have to have an operation   _____   _____

39. Having a sudden hospitalization you weren't planning to have   _____   _____

40. Knowing you have a serious illness   _____   _____

41. Thinking you might lose a kidney or some other organ   _____   _____

42. Thinking you might have cancer   _____   _____

Separation from Family

43. Being in the hospital during holidays or special occasions   _____   _____

44. Not having family visit you   _____   _____

45. Being hospitalized far away from home   _____   _____

Problems with Medications

46. Having medications cause you discomfort   _____   _____

47. Feeling you are becoming dependent on medications   _____   _____

48. Not getting relief from pain medications   _____   _____

49. Not getting pain medication when you need it   _____   _____

Scoring the HSRS

The mean values for each hospital event are listed below. Write in the mean values for those events that you checked as being of significant concern or stressful.

Event	Value	Event	Value	Event	Value
1	14	17	29	33	32
2	16	18	41	34	34
3	17	19	23	35	34
4	17	20	28	36	22
5	19	21	26	37	27
6	22	22	27	38	27
7	23	23	21	39	27
8	23	24	22	40	35
9	15	25	22	41	36
10	16	26	23	42	39
11	17	27	25	43	22
12	18	28	35	44	27
13	18	29	22	45	27
14	19	30	24	46	26
15	22	31	26	47	26
16	27	32	28	48	31
				49	32

Your overall level of "hospital stress" can be determined by adding all mean values for the events that you checked. After adding all of the mean values, record your total hospital stress score on the HSRS scoring table that follows. You also can determine your level of stress for each of the separate hospital-related factors by adding the mean values of the items you checked in each section separately. For example, if you checked number 1, 4, and 5 listed under the Unfamiliarity of Surroundings section, then your score for that section would be 50 (14+17+19). For each of the nine sections, add up your mean value scores and record the results in the HSRS scoring table.

The average score column will help you interpret your score as compared to other surgery patients. The average scores in the chart below are from the 250 surgical patients in Dr. Volicer's research study.

HSRS Scoring Table

	Average Score	Your Score
Total Hospital Stress	290	_____
Unfamiliarity of Surroundings	55	_____
Loss of Independence	68	_____
Separation from Spouse or Significant Other	23	_____
Financial Problems	8	_____
Isolation from Other People	11	_____
Lack of Information	40	_____
Threat of Severe Illness	62	_____
Separation from Family	9	_____
Problems with Medications	14	_____

* Hospital Stress Rating Scale. Reprinted from *Journal of Human Stress,* June 1977, B. J. Volicer, M. A. Isenberg and M. W. Burns, "Medical-Surgical Differences in Hospital Stress Factors," page 7, copyright 1977, with permission from Heldref Publications, Washington, D.C.

Coping

People respond to stress in individual ways by using different types of "coping strategies." Your coping strategies are elicited when you appraise a situation as stressful or threatening. They are your attempt to decrease the stress associated with the threatening situation. Examples of coping strategies might include such responses as trying to focus on positive aspects of the situation, expressing emotions, gaining support from family and friends, or denying the stress altogether. The particular type of coping strategies that you use will depend upon your personality characteristics, your social and family situation, and the nature of the stress you experience.

The following questionnaire helps you to assess the coping strategies you are most likely to use. This information is an essential part of the preparation for surgery program and helps you to choose healthy rather than unhealthy coping strategies.

Ways of Coping Scale-Revised*

Instructions: Please read the following list of things people do in reaction to their medical condition and/or undergoing surgery and hospitalization. Please indicate whether you have ever done any of these things in reaction to your medical condition or a previous surgery, hospitalization, or stressful medical procedure. Rate each item according to the following scale.

0 = Never have done it
1 = Done it on a seldom basis
2 = Done it sometimes

3 = Done it often
4 = Do it most of the time

Changing Thoughts

1. Concentrated on something good that could come out of the whole thing	0	1	2	3	4
2. Rediscover what is important in life	0	1	2	3	4
3. Felt like you changed or grew as a person in a good way	0	1	2	3	4
4. Found new faith or some truth about life	0	1	2	3	4
5. Remembered times when your life was more difficult	0	1	2	3	4
6. Religion became more important	0	1	2	3	4
7. Thought about people who were worse off than you	0	1	2	3	4
8. Reminded yourself that things could be worse	0	1	2	3	4
9. Looked for the silver lining, so to speak; tried to look on the bright side of things	0	1	2	3	4
10. Did something totally new that you never would have done if this hadn't happened	0	1	2	3	4
11. Changed the way you did things so that the illness was less of a problem	0	1	2	3	4
12. Got away from it for a while; tried to rest or take a vacation	0	1	2	3	4

Emotional Expression

1. Took it out on other people	0	1	2	3	4
2. Got help with day-to-day chores or travel	0	1	2	3	4
3. Joked about it	0	1	2	3	4
4. Let your feelings out somehow	0	1	2	3	4
5. Avoided being with people in general	0	1	2	3	4
6. Recalled past successes	0	1	2	3	4
7. Daydreamed or imagined a better time or place than the one you were in	0	1	2	3	4
8. Slept more than usual	0	1	2	3	4

Fantasizing

1. Wished that you could change what happened	0	1	2	3	4
2. Wished that you could change the way you felt	0	1	2	3	4
3. Felt bad that you couldn't avoid the problem	0	1	2	3	4
4. Wished that the situation would go away or somehow be over with	0	1	2	3	4
5. Hoped a miracle would happen	0	1	2	3	4
6. Wished you were a stronger person	0	1	2	3	4
7. Had fantasies or wishes about how things might turn out	0	1	2	3	4

Self-Blame

1. Blamed yourself	0	1	2	3	4

2. Thought about fantastic or unreal things that made you feel better	0	1	2	3	4
3. Saw the doctor and did what he or she recommended	0	1	2	3	4
4. Got mad at the people or things that caused the problem	0	1	2	3	4
5. Criticized or took it out on yourself	0	1	2	3	4
6. Realized you brought the problem on yourself	0	1	2	3	4
7. Refused to believe it had happened					

Seeking Information

1. Looked up medical information	0	1	2	3	4
2. Read books or magazine articles (or watched TV) about your medical condition or surgery	0	1	2	3	4
3. Came up with some different solutions to the problem	0	1	2	3	4
4. Asked someone other than your doctor you respected for advice and followed it	0	1	2	3	4
5. Made a plan of action and followed it	0	1	2	3	4

Minimizing the Threat

1. Kept your feelings to yourself	0	1	2	3	4
2. Went on as if nothing had happened	0	1	2	3	4
3. Talked to someone about how you were feeling	0	1	2	3	4
4. Didn't let it get to you; refused to think too much about it	0	1	2	3	4
5. Kept others from knowing how bad things were	0	1	2	3	4
6. Tried to forget the whole thing	0	1	2	3	4

7. Talked to someone other than a doctor who could do something about the problem for you	0	1	2	3	4
8. Tried to work it out by yourself	0	1	2	3	4
9. Accepted sympathy and understanding from someone	0	1	2	3	4
10. Made light of the situation; refused to get too serious about it	0	1	2	3	4
11. Went along with fate; sometimes you just have bad luck	0	1	2	3	4

Scoring the Ways of Coping Scale

The six sections of the Ways of Coping Scale can be scored separately. First, add the total for each section and record the number in the Ways of Coping Scoring Table under the heading "Total Score." Next, divide that number by the number of items in the section (this is the number under the heading "Divide by"). This will give an average score for that type of coping strategy. Record this number under the heading "Average."

Ways of Coping Scoring Table

Section	Total Score	Divide by:	Average
Changing Thoughts	_____	12	_____
Emotional Expression	_____	8	_____
Fantasizing	_____	7	_____
Self-Blame	_____	7	_____
Seeking Information	_____	5	_____
Minimizing the Threat	_____	11	_____

Summary Sheet

The following lists summarize all the information you have collected about yourself that you can use to design your preparation for surgery program. Please transfer your results to the page below for use throughout the remainder of this book.

Degree of Depression: _____

Degree of Anxiety: _____

Degree of Anger: _____

Summary of Hospital Stress from the Hospital Stress Rating Scale

Circle each of the following scales for which your score was above average. Each circled area represents a source of probable stress to be addressed in the preparation program.

Total Hospital Stress	Above Average
Unfamiliarity of Surroundings	Above Average
Loss of Independence	Above Average
Separation from Spouse	Above Average
Financial Problems	Above Average
Isolation from Other People	Above Average
Lack of Information	Above Average
Threat of Severe Illness	Above Average
Separation from Family	Above Average
Problems with Medications	Above Average

Ways of Coping Scale Summary

For each of the following coping areas, transfer your average score from the Ways of Coping Scoring Table. This information will be used later to assess your coping strategies and to develop a healthy approach to coping.

Section   *Average*

Changing Thoughts   _____

Emotional Expression   _____

Fantasizing   _____

Self-Blame   _____

Seeking Information   _____

Minimizing the Threat   _____

Using Your Questionnaire Results

The results of your questionnaires, as listed in the Summary Sheet, will help you to choose the most appropriate and effective techniques in the design of your preparation for surgery program. Refer to them as you progress through this book. The following brief overview suggests ways in which these results may be applied to your program.

Depression, Anxiety, and Anger

The experience of high, or even moderate, levels of depression, anxiety, or anger can have a negative impact on your surgery and recovery. It is important that you address the sources of these emotions as part of your preparation for surgery program. The cognitive exercises in Chapters 5 and 6 can be very helpful in changing the thoughts that cause these emotions. The chapters concerning spirituality, affirmations, assertiveness, and communication can be very effective in helping to manage anger. Keep in mind your Degrees of Depression, Anxiety, and Anger as recorded in the Summary Sheet.

Hospital Stress

The results of the hospital stress rating scale, as shown in the Summary Sheet, can help you prepare to cope with those aspects of the hospital environment that may be stressful for you. Of course, this is different for everyone. For instance, if your scores are above average in the categories of Loss of Independence and Separation from Family, you might focus on these issues when developing your coping strategies and relaxation exercises. You might also plan ahead by determining what the hospital visiting hours are, and how your family members will schedule their time with you. Your concern over the loss of your independence might be addressed by practicing the assertiveness and communication techniques in Chapter 12. If lack of information is a high concern, you might consider more detailed answers to the questions presented in Chapter 3. These are just a few examples of how to use the results of the HSRS in designing your program.

Your Coping Style

The Ways of Coping Scale Summary provides information about how you tend to cope with stressful situations. If you scored high in the Changing Thoughts section, then you may be very comfortable with the cognitive techniques in Chapters 5 and 6. On the other hand, if your score was very low in this section, then these cognitive techniques may initially seem difficult. In any case, it is important that you learn these strategies as they are essential to the surgical coping and recovery process.

A high score on the Emotional Expression section might indicate that you are prone to "take it out on others" or to withdraw. Awareness of this pattern can help you avoid it through use of cognitive, relaxation, and assertiveness techniques.

Excessive fantasizing or a tendency towards self-blame can be destructive, especially under stress. Using specific guided imagery can help you to develop "healthy" fantasies. You may employ affirmations and challenge negative thoughts to decrease self-blame.

If you scored high in the area of seeking information, you may be likely to cope with a stressful situation by collecting as much detailed information as possible. Pay particular attention to the questions in the next chapter as well as the resources in the appendices.

If you tend to minimize the threat, collecting detailed information may not benefit you. If you scored high in this area, collect only as much information as you feel comfortable with. Also, the strategies of distraction and focusing on other aspects of your life may be effective.

3

Gathering Information About Your Surgery: Taking an Active Role

After completing the assessments in the previous chapter, you will have a lot of good information about your emotional state and the issues that need to be addressed as part of your preparation for surgery program. This chapter is another exercise in gathering important information about your surgery and recovery to ensure that you have adequate information about:

- Surgical decision making

- The details of your surgery

- What to do before the surgery

- What to expect and do after the surgery

- What to expect during your hospitalization

Understanding and Remembering Medical Information

When helping to prepare patients for surgery, we often find that they actually know little about the nature and purpose of the operation being planned. Research consistently shows that patients are often dissatisfied with the medical information they receive, and so have poor understanding and recall of that information.

How Well Do People Understand and Remember What They Are Told by Their Doctor?

Many patients have a poor understanding of the medical information presented to them and remember little of what they are told. Medical forms are often complex. Many surgical consent forms are written at the level of scientific journals, beyond the comprehension of most people. Not surprisingly, only about 40 percent or less of patients read them carefully.

Patients can become frustrated in their attempts to get understandable information from their doctors. As a result, they have questions they don't ask and desire more information than they are given.

Retention of information about surgery is another problem. Patients remember 30 percent to 50 percent of the simple verbal information they are given about surgery and only slightly more when it is written.

Inadequate comprehension and memory of information about surgery frequently leads to patient dissatisfaction with communication and can compromise overall treatment.

Bernard was scheduled to undergo hip replacement surgery and was referred for a brief mind-body preparation for surgery program. In the initial evaluation, we asked him about his understanding of the surgery (questions similar to those contained in this chapter). Bernard's case was dramatic in that he could answer virtually none of the questions even though his surgery was only two weeks away. He wasn't sure which hospital was scheduled for the surgery and couldn't relate any details about the surgery or the postoperative rehabilitation. It became evident that his lack of information was due to two factors. He was afraid to question his doctors and he was too nervous to remember what he was told. The preparation for surgery program helped Bernard learn how to acquire, understand, and remember the information he needed.

A good understanding of the surgery and related procedures can improve your outcome and make surgery a less stressful experience. Information can be obtained from several sources including your surgeon, family doctor, patient education brochures, the hospital, and your insurance company. Some other suggested sources of information will be provided throughout this chapter.

The following questions about your surgery developed from our preparation for surgery program as well as from the resources listed in the References and Resources section at the end of the book. Ask your surgeon, doctor, or other healthcare professional these questions, get clear answers, and write them down in the spaces provided. You may want to take someone with you on your presurgical doctor visits.

Surgical Decision Making

What is wrong with me? What is my diagnosis?

You should have a sufficient understanding of your diagnosis to be able to express it in your own words. Also, knowing your exact diagnosis is important when you talk with different doctors who don't know you well and who may not have previous medical records readily available. It is a good idea to write down your diagnosis.

_____

_____

_____

_____

Why do I need the surgery?

_____

_____

_____

_____

How will the surgery improve my condition?

Surgery is done with the goal of curing a medical condition (e.g., gallbladder, tonsil, or appendix removal), improving the quality of life (e.g., joint replacement, back surgery to relieve pain), or extending life (e.g., removing a cancerous tumor). You should find out exactly how your surgery is expected to help you.

_____

_____

_____

_____

What other treatment options are available and have they been successful?

You should feel sure that appropriate nonsurgical treatment methods have been attempted and that surgery is the best choice for your condition.

_____

_____

_____

_____

_____

What will happen if I decline the surgery or delay it until a later date? How long can I safely delay the surgery?

Most surgeries are elective and the scheduling of the operation is somewhat flexible. Therefore, when you schedule your surgery you may want to consider job and family commitments, the surgeon's schedule, and time to prepare for the operation, among other matters.

_____

_____

_____

_____

_____

What are the risks of the surgery? Do the benefits of the surgery outweigh the risks?

All the possible risks of a surgical procedure will usually be presented to you in written form on an informed consent sheet. You will be required to sign this prior to the surgery. This information is often presented in a legal format which can be intimidating and difficult to understand. You should discuss risks and benefits with your surgeon as you make decisions about your surgery.

_____

_____

_____

_____

If the surgery is successful, what results can I expect? If it is unsuccessful (or only partially successful), what remaining symptoms can I expect and what are my treatment options?

Many patients have unrealistic expectations and are disappointed about the outcome of their surgery even though it was a "technical" success. Some surgeries are designed to reduce pain or improve functioning but not to "cure" the problem. If the patient expects a "cure" but is only somewhat improved, the postoperative recovery may be made more difficult by unmet expectations.

We once worked with a woman who, one month after her operation, was very distressed about her ongoing "strange" physical symptoms, including numbness in her arms, heaviness in her legs and feet, and "feeling big all over." She had had extensive surgery to remove a spinal tumor in the area of her neck. Even though it was a very serious medical condition, the tumor was discovered before the patient had any real physical symptoms. The surgery was a technical success. Removal of the tumor left her physical abilities almost completely intact. Still, she expressed great distress and depression because she had experienced no symptoms prior to surgery, but after surgery had symptoms she neither understood nor expected. Had she been given realistic expectations prior to surgery about these possible symptoms, her postoperative coping could have been greatly enhanced.

_____

_____

_____

_____

_____

The Details of Your Surgery

If you are an information-seeker and want more information on your particular surgery, two excellent resources are the books by Dr. Macho and Dr. Youngson listed in the References and Resources section for Chapter 1.

Can you describe the surgery to me in simple language?

You should have a general understanding of the nature of your surgical procedure, although detailed knowledge may not be helpful to you. It is important that you be able to explain, in your own words, what the surgery will entail. Consider your answers to these questions depending on whether you are an information-seeker or information-avoider.

_____

_____

_____

_____

_____

Do you have a brochure or information sheet that describes the surgery?   YES   NO

If not, do you know where I can obtain a bro-chure, written for laypeople, that describes the procedure?   YES   NO

_____

_____

How will I feel immediately after the surgery in the recovery room?

Research has shown that patients who are well-informed about the physical sensations they may expect following surgery adjust better to the recovery period. You should be told what you will feel, hear, smell, taste, and see before, during, and after the procedure. Many questions in this section address this issue. Record the answer to the question above on the lines below.

_____

_____

_____

_____

_____

How long can I expect to be hospitalized? How can I expect to feel, what will I be able to do, and what should I try and do, each day in the hospital after the surgery?

It is important to know beforehand what kind of physical sensations you can expect as your body heals from the surgery. These may include pain, nausea, numbness, tingling, itching, etc., in certain areas of your body (especially with specific movements); shortness of breath or dizziness; or difficulty in urinating or walking.

The specific symptoms you might experience after surgery will depend on your condition and the nature of your surgery. If you know what kind of sensations to expect after your surgery, you will not be worried or fearful when they occur. This will help to decrease your overall suffering and increase your sense of control. It is also helpful to know what will be expected from you as you recover. For instance, you may be required to get out of bed and walk fairly soon after surgery or to do certain exercises. Record below how you will be expected to feel and what you will be expected to do as part of your recovery.

Day One

_____

Day Two

_____

Day Three

_____

Day Four

_____

Day Five

_____

Day Six

_____

Day Seven

_____

(Make any necessary additions on a separate piece of paper.)

What complications might arise after surgery or after being discharged from the hospital? What is the best way to manage these complications if they arise? With whom should I discuss these issues?

During your surgery and recovery, several professionals may take care of you, including doctors, nurses, physician's assistants, respiratory therapists, physical therapists, and others. This can be quite confusing and overwhelming if you have questions to ask. Consider that the answers to some questions may not be known prior to surgery.

_____

_____

_____

_____

_____

Will I need assistance at home after I am discharged from the hospital? Should I arrange for that now? Will I go directly home after discharge or is it possible that I may go to a rehabilitation or transitional care facility? Will I need any medical supplies at home?

Depending on your medical condition and the type of surgery you are undergoing, you may need a period of professional assistance at home (home nursing) or to be transferred to another type of treatment setting (transitional unit or hospital) for extended postoperative care. However, this is more often the case for the elderly or those with medical complications. It is very helpful to know about this possibility beforehand.

_____

_____

_____

_____

Once I go home, how will my level of functioning be limited and for how long?

It is useful to know how much bed rest you will need and the extent and duration of any physical limitations you may experience. If there is an extended postoperative phase with significant physical limitations, you can plan ahead by doing such things as getting materials together for your diversion (videotapes, books, etc.), arranging for food and other necessary items, and organizing help and visitation from family and friends.

_____

_____

_____

_____

Blood Transfusion

A "blood transfusion" is the medical term for receiving blood. In most planned surgeries patients lose such a small amount of blood that transfusions are not necessary. Examples of surgeries that may require you to have a blood transfusion include the following:

- Orthopedic

- Cardiac

- Chest surgery

- Gynecological (a woman's reproductive system)

- Blood vessel surgery

- Other major surgeries

There are basically three ways to prepare for blood transfusion:

Autologous Blood Donation. In this procedure you donate your own blood prior to surgery. You can give one unit of blood per week for up to about six weeks depending on the amount needed. A "unit" of blood is just under one pint and is about 10 percent of the total blood supply in an adult. A healthy person can normally regenerate this much blood in about three days. The last donation of blood is usually made no later than three days before surgery. Autologous blood donation is the safest procedure and has the lowest risk of infectious disease transmission and those transfusion reactions that may result from receiving another donor's blood. Also, the process of donating your own blood prior to surgery stimulates the production of blood cells in the bone marrow, so that your body will more rapidly replace the blood lost during surgery.

Homologous Blood Donation. In this type of blood donation, the blood provided is to be used by someone other than the donor. Blood from the public supply (a blood bank) comes from homologous blood donations. The current community blood supply is as safe as it has ever been and there are currently more types of blood screening tests than ever before. Even so, donating your own blood prior to surgery is considered the safest method, but if time does not permit that, or if the surgery is an emergency, using the blood bank is certainly a wise decision entailing very little risk.

Checking Up on Your Doctor and Avoiding Medical Errors

The Journal of the American Medical Association estimates that mistakes made by doctors or hospitals could be at least partially related to 180,000 deaths annually! Many medical errors are preventable, and there are steps you can take to protect yourself.

First, check up on your doctor. Call the state medical-licensing board to find out if any complaints have been made. Determine if a doctor is board-certified by calling the American Board of Medical Specialties in Evanston, IL. (800-776-CERT). If you have trouble finding the correct agency contact the People's Medical Society, 462 Walnut St., Allentown, PA 18102 (610-770-1670).

Second, make sure your doctor is willing to keep you well informed about your medical condition and treatment. Also, be a responsible partner in your own treatment by taking an active role. Know your medical history, the names of your medicines, and other important information about your health.

Third, and most importantly, speak up and ask questions. This is the best weapon you have to protect yourself from medical errors.

Autotransfusion. This process is generally used when it is anticipated that a very large amount of blood will be lost during the surgery. Autotransfusion devices collect the patient's own blood during the operation and return it to the body. This type of procedure is often done during very complicated and lengthy surgeries.

In summary, issues related to blood donation to be aware of include the following:

- A unit of blood is just under one pint.

- A person has about ten units of blood. A healthy person can quickly recover from the 10-percent-blood-volume loss associated with donating a unit of blood.

- Although patients can donate blood every three days, once a week is the most common frequency for autologous donation purposes.

- Liquid blood cells can be stored for up to forty-two days.

- In autologous blood collection the last donation is usually done no later than seventy-two hours before surgery.

You generally have the option of getting blood from a blood bank or from friends and relatives, or of using your own blood. If the blood comes from you or your friends and relatives, it will be donated prior to the surgery and stored for later use. Liquid blood can be stored for about forty-two days. If blood will be required for your surgery, the following questions will help you to prepare adequately. Circle one-word answers and write longer answers in the space provided.

Is it possible that I may need a blood transfusion during the surgery?   YES   NO

Can I give blood in advance in case I need it during the surgery?   YES   NO

Where should I go to give blood before my operation? Record below the address, phone number, and contact person at the blood collection center.

_____

_____

_____

_____

Is there enough time before surgery to give the blood that I may need?

As discussed above, there is a limit to how quickly you can give your own blood for surgery. Should you decide to use your own blood, be sure there is enough time before your surgery to provide an adequate supply. List below the dates for your own blood donations.

_____

_____

_____

_____

_____

What to Do Before the Surgery

What presurgical tests or evaluations are necessary? Who will be doing these and when should they be done?

You may need a presurgical/preadmission medical evaluation, especially if you are undergoing general anesthesia. This includes evaluation of your heart (electrocardiogram), lungs (chest X rays), and kidneys (urinalysis). Your presurgical medical evaluation might also include blood tests to assess for infection, clotting time, and other things. This evaluation might be done by your family doctor or another physician. Find out from your surgeon which doctor will be responsible for this presurgical/preadmission evaluation.

_____

_____

_____

_____

_____

Should I make sure my family physician knows about the surgery?

Yes   Not Necessary   Notified on: _____

Will my family doctor be involved in my postoperative care? Does he or she need any special medical records?

In this age of managed care, you must assume more responsibility to see that you get good care. This responsibility includes helping to coordinate the roles of the various doctors involved. If they need medical records, it may be most efficient to get them yourself. Many doctors' offices and hospitals are slow in sending records to outside sources. We highly recommend that your family physician should be provided with copies of all your medical records.

_____

_____

_____

_____

_____

Do I need to be on a special diet before or after the surgery? If so, can you explain it in detail?

_____

_____

_____

_____

Questions About the Hospitalization

**Will this operation be done on an outpatient   Outpatient   Inpatient
or inpatient basis?**

In what hospital will the operation be done?
        Record the address, general directions, and phone number below.

_____

_____

_____

Are the surgery and hospitalization preapproved by the insurance company?
        The answer to this question will come from several sources including your doctor's office, the hospital admitting department, and your insurance company.

Exact Procedure Approved: _____

_____

Date of Approval: _____

Have you received a copy of the   YES   NO
hospitalization approval letter from
insurance company?

Number of hospitalization days preapproved by the insurance company: _____

What if my surgeon recommends a longer hospitalization than has been approved? How do I get approval and who can assist me?

We often hear horror stories from patients about insurance coverage issues. Usually the patient believes a procedure or charge is covered only to find, after the fact, that it is not. Dr. Deardorff experienced this when his wife underwent a Caesarean section with a three-day "preapproved" hospital stay. Due to a high fever, her doctor kept her in the hospital for a fourth day with clearly documented medical reasons. The insurance company denied coverage for the fourth day retroactively and attempted to collect the entire charge for that day (a very significant amount). After two years of correspondence and phone conversation with the insurance company and hospital, the charges were finally covered.

Get very specific information on this issue prior to the surgery. Do not rely on your doctor's office or the hospital to see that coverage is adequate.

_____

_____

_____

_____

_____

Phone contact Log with the hospital and insurance company about coverage:

Since you are ultimately financially responsible for your medical bills, we have found that it is very important to document discussions about insurance coverage and reimbursement issues. A phone contact log provides a means of keeping track of conversations in case problems arise at a later date.

Name of Person	*Date and Time*	*Topic*

_____

_____

What doctors can I expect to see in the hospital and what are their roles?

Many doctors may be involved in your treatment depending on the nature of your surgery and other medical problems. It can be helpful to know what specialists may assist in your care and whether you should see a particular doctor again after you are discharged. Prior to surgery you may not know all the doctors who will be involved in your care, so don't be afraid to ask for each doctor's business card. We have found that by keeping the cards in an inexpensive, plastic business-card notebook you will be able to find them when you need them.

Doctor	*Office Phone*	*Specialty/Purpose*	*Follow-up After Discharge*	
			YES	NO
			YES	NO
			YES	NO
			YES	NO
			YES	NO

When will I first see my surgeon in the hospital after the surgery?

Ask about this in advance.

_____

_____

_____

Will my surgeon be in town and managing my case the entire time I am in the hospital?

Your surgeon may plan to be out of town or on vacation immediately following your surgery. It can be distressing to have another doctor manage your postoperative recovery if you are not expecting it. Ask about this and make contact with the backup physician prior to the surgery if necessary.

_____

_____

_____

Pain Control

The issue of pain control is so important that we have devoted an entire chapter to it. See Chapter 4 for information about pain-control procedures and relevant questions to ask.

Your Relationship with Your Doctor

Your relationships with your doctor and surgeon are extremely important. A good relationship or partnership with your doctor improves the overall quality of care and your response to treatment. It helps make you more comfortable in taking an active role in your preparation for surgery.

The Trust in Physician Scale (TPS) was developed by Dr. Lynda Anderson to assess a patient's trust in his or her physician (Anderson and Dedrick 1990).

Trust-in-Physician Scale (TPS)*

Each item below is a statement with which you may agree or disagree. Beside each statement is a scale that ranges from "Strongly agree" (1) to "Strongly disagree" (5). For each item circle the number that represents the extent to which you agree or disagree with the statement.

Make sure that you answer every item and that you circle only one number per item. It is important that you respond according to what you actually believe, and not according to what you feel you should believe.

1 = Strongly agree   4 = Disagree
2 = Agree   5 = Strongly disagree
3 = Neutral

Checking Up on Your Hospital and Taking Charge

The Joint Commission on Accreditation of Healthcare Organizations (JCAHO) is the agency that determines whether a hospital meets specific standards of care. To determine if a hospital is accredited call JCAHO (708-916-5800). You can also get a "report card" on a particular hospital from this agency.

Even JCAHO accreditation does not mean you shouldn't take steps to protect yourself while hospitalized. For example, in about 12 percent of all medications administered in hospitals, there are errors; including not getting a medication on schedule, getting the wrong medication, or getting medication that causes an allergic reaction or other negative interactions with other medicines (Austin 1995). You should keep track of the medicines you are given and alert the nurse of any changes or reactions.

Being in the hospital is stressful. One of the best means for avoiding mistakes is to have a family member or friend act as your advocate who can ask questions and help you through your experience. If you do experience problems in the hospital that are not easily resolved with the staff, you can contact the hospital's patient representative for assistance.

1. I doubt that my doctor really cares about me as a person.   1   2   3   4   5

2. My doctor is usually considerate of my needs and puts them first.   1   2   3   4   5

3. I trust my doctor so much that I will always follow her/his advice regarding my medical condition.   1   2   3   4   5

4. If my doctor tells me something is so, then it must be true.   1   2   3   4   5

5. I sometimes mistrust my doctor's opinion about my condition and would like a second one.   1   2   3   4   5

6. I trust my doctor's judgments about my medical care.   1   2   3   4   5

7. I feel my doctor does not do everything he/she should for my medical care.   1   2   3   4   5

8. I trust my doctor to put my medical needs above all other considerations when treating my medical problems.   1   2   3   4   5

9. My doctor is a real expert in taking care of medical problems like mine.   1   2   3   4   5

10. I trust my doctor to tell me if a mistake was made about my treatment.   1   2   3   4   5

11. I sometimes worry that my doctor may not keep the information we discuss totally private.   1   2   3   4   5

To score the TPS, items 1, 5, 7, and 11 are reversed scored. For those items you score the exact opposite of what you marked. For example, if you circled a 1 that would count as 5; if you circled a 2, that would count as 4; and if you circled a 3, that remains a 3. All other items are simply scored at the number value that you marked. Score each question and add the total number of items after reverse-scoring items 1, 5, 7, and 11. A higher score reflects greater trust in your treating professional. In the research sample studied, the average was approximately 48.

* Reproduced with permission of authors and publisher from: L. A. Anderson, and R. F. Dedrick, "Development of the Trust in Physician Scale: a Measure to Assess Interpersonal Trust in Patient-Physician Relationships." *Psychological Reports*, 1990, 67, 1091-1100.

A good, trusting relationship with your doctor is very important to the successful outcome of your treatment. Even so, we must also emphasize that "blind trust" is not a healthy way to approach your surgery. You should have a high level of trust in your treating professionals, while also retaining some skepticism about their recommendations. Above all, you should be able to question your doctor and get the information you need.

Making Your Own Medical Fact Sheet

In addition to getting the answers to the questions discussed in this chapter, it can be useful to design your own medical fact sheet. This sheet (or sheets) presents information about your medical status and history in a summarized and concise manner. It should include (but not be limited to) such categories as:

- Daily medications

- As-needed medications

- Allergies

- A list of all your doctors

- A list of all your previous surgeries and medical problems

- Any other important information

How Does Being Assertive Affect Your Relationship with Your Doctor?

Research has shown the effects of teaching patients to be more assertive in getting information from their doctors. In one study, patients were given ten-minute sessions prior to visits with their doctors in which they were taught how to ask questions about their medical condition and treatment. Results indicated that these patients asked more questions, were more willing to keep future doctor's appointments, and felt more in control of their health condition as compared to patients who did not receive the training. (Roter 1977).

Even with these positive benefits there were some problems. As the patients became more assertive, the doctor-patient interaction was rated as more distressful overall, and patients were found to be less satisfied with their doctor visits.

Given these results, an approach that balances assertiveness with respect for the doctor's time is most effective. This balanced approach is presented in Chapter 12.

Give this handout to any new doctors you see, take it with you to the hospital to be placed in your surgical/medical chart, and keep it at your hospital bedside. It can help your doctors and nurses avoid mistakes such as giving you the wrong medicines, not knowing about your other medical conditions, and so forth.

An example of a medical fact sheet follows. There is also a checklist of things to have ready before you go to the hospital.

DETAILED MEDICAL FACT SHEET

NAME _____

ADDRESS _____

_____

TELEPHONE _____

MALE/FEMALE   BIRTH DATE _____ AGE _____

EMERGENCY CONTACT _____

TELEPHONE _____

SPECIAL PROBLEMS (HEARING, MOVEMENT, VISION, ETC.) _____

_____

CURRENT MEDICAL CONDITIONS   **EXPLANATION**

_____ Shortness of breath   _____

_____ High blood pressure   _____

_____ Chest pains   _____

_____ Diabetes   _____

_____ Asthma   _____

_____ Impaired immunity   _____

_____ Liver disease   _____

_____ Kidney disease   _____

_____ Infections   _____

_____ Paralysis or stroke   _____

NAME _____

_____ Convulsions   _____

_____ Dizziness   _____

_____ Memory loss   _____

_____ Depression   _____

_____ Chronic anxiety   _____

_____ Weight loss   _____

_____ Weight gain   _____

_____ Heart disease   _____

_____ Blood vessel disease _____

_____ Back problems   _____

_____ Pain conditions   _____

_____ Headaches   _____

_____ Bleeding conditions _____

_____ Thyroid problems   _____

_____ Pain medications   _____

_____ Drug/substance use   _____

_____ Alcohol abuse   _____

_____ Smoking   _____

_____ Other   _____

                           _____

                           _____

NAME _____   Page 3

PAST MEDICAL CONDITIONS   EXPLANATION/DATES

_____ Rheumatic fever   _____

_____ Tuberculosis   _____

_____ Hepatitis   _____

_____ Other infections   _____

_____ Seizures/convulsions _____

_____ Cancer   _____

_____ Stroke   _____

_____ Heart attack   _____

_____ Other   _____

                                _____

_____ Treatment with cortisone or similar medications _____

                                _____

_____ Treatment with chemotherapy _____

                                _____

_____ Smoking history   _____

_____ Alcohol use/abuse   _____

                                _____

_____ Substance abuse history _____

                                _____

NAME _____   Page 4

SURGERY HISTORY

On the following pages record the history of your surgeries, the dates, your age at the time of the surgery, the type of anesthesia used, and any problems that may have occurred. Types of anesthesia include general, regional (spinal, epidural), and local.

Date	Surgery	Age	Type of Anesthesia	Complications?

Current Medications	Dose	Amount Taken Per Day	/	Time	/	Side Effects

NAME _____

ALLERGIC REACTIONS TO MEDICATIONS

Medication   *Type of Reactions*

_____

_____

_____

_____

_____

_____

PHYSICIANS AND SPECIALISTS INVOLVED IN YOUR MEDICAL CARE

Family Physician _____ Dates of Treatment _____

Name   _____

Address   _____

_____

Telephone _____ Fax _____

Speciality _____ Dates of Treatment _____

Name   _____

Address   _____

_____

Telephone _____ Fax _____

NAME _____   Page 6

Speciality _____ Dates of Treatment _____

Name   _____

Address   _____

_____

Telephone _____ Fax _____

Speciality _____ Dates of Treatment _____

Name   _____

Address   _____

_____

Telephone _____ Fax _____

Speciality _____ Dates of Treatment _____

Name   _____

Address   _____

_____

Telephone _____ Fax _____

Speciality _____ Dates of Treatment _____

Name   _____

Address   _____

_____

Telephone _____ Fax _____

Hospital Checklist

1. Scheduling and Approvals

_____ Do you have your insurance preapproval letter?

_____ Has your insurance deductible been met?

_____ Do you know how much your copayment will be?

_____ Does your employer know about the time you will need off from work?

2. Preoperative procedures

_____ Are all of the preoperative procedures completed (lab and blood tests, internal medicine evaluation, etc.)?

_____ Does your surgeon have all of your necessary records?

_____ Do you have copies of important records (or the completed medical fact sheet)?

_____ Do you need a sedative for the night before?

_____ Do you need to rent any special equipment for recovery at home?

_____ Are "advanced directives" (living will or durable power of attorney for health care) completed if you desire them?

_____ Are presurgical instructions understood and completed (e.g., no food or liquid twenty-four hours before, bowel preparation, etc.)?

_____ Is an interpreter service arranged if necessary?

3. Bring to the hospital

_____ Your insurance card

_____ Pajamas or nightgown, robe, slippers, appropriate clothes, toiletries

_____ List of medications

_____ Completed medical fact sheet (3 copies)

_____ Your plastic business-card notebook

_____ Reading/inspirational materials (if desired)

_____ Notepad and pencil

4. Do not bring valuables to the hospital

5. Other

_____

_____

_____

_____

PART II

Managing the Pain of Surgery

Pain is an inevitable part of surgery and it is also one of the most feared consequences of surgery. Unabated, pain can profoundly affect surgical recovery, but recent advances in pain control have markedly reduced the amount of postsurgical pain. Understanding your pain control options is an important step in preparing for surgery and enhancing recovery.

The purpose of Part II is to provide you with guidelines to discuss pain control options with your surgeon and surgical team and to design with them a mutually agreeable surgical pain management plan. This chapter will help you to understand the following:

- What pain is as well as its physical and emotional impact on surgical recovery

- What questions to ask your surgeon and surgical team about pain control

- What your pain control options are

- How to communicate your pain to the surgical team

- How to develop a pain control strategy before, during, and after surgery with your surgeon and surgical team

4

Pain Control

Pain is an experience both universal and unique. You can't see, hear, touch, or otherwise perceive another person's pain directly. No wonder pain has mystified people since humankind's beginnings.

—Cindy Rippa

What Is Pain?

Pain is a profoundly distasteful experience for most of us, but it is also a mechanism for protection. Typically, pain signals that something is wrong. It immediately commands our attention, disrupts our activities, and strikes at the core of our emotional being. Without the capacity to feel pain, however, we would not survive very long. For example, failure to feel the severe abdominal pain of a ruptured appendix can be fatal. Thus, pain is both physically and emotionally disruptive and at the same time it is a useful signal that something is wrong that must be attended to.

The human nervous system is well adapted to register pain. Throughout our bodies we have specialized pain receptors that act as entry points or terminals for pain messages. When these terminals are stimulated by a trauma, a complicated series of chemical events send a pain message along specialized nerves into the spinal cord. The pain message is processed and interpreted at specific control centers in the spinal cord before it is sent to the brain. When the pain message enters the brain it undergoes amazing transformations. The brain, which contains all of our current and past experiences, thoughts, and emotions, interprets the pain message and gives it meaning. The brain, in turn, sends messages back down the spinal cord to the control centers and to the areas of injury, where it may modify the pain messages being sent to it from the injured site.

As can be seen, there is a complex interplay between the site of injury, the spinal cord, and the brain that is established from the moment of injury. The brain orchestrates this interplay of information and actually creates the experience of pain. This is based not only on the pain messages sent to it through the nervous system, but also on our personal history of life experiences, our emotional status, our psychological coping resources, our prior experiences with pain, and the meaning and context of the pain. Because we all have very different life experiences stored in our brains, we experience pain in unique and deeply personal ways. This is why we vary greatly in our perception of pain, our reports of pain, our ability to tolerate it, and in our need for pain medications. Some of us suffer greatly, while others seem to suffer very little, if at all. Certainly, the mind-body connection is exemplified by our response to pain and our ability to cope with it.

Surgical Pain: The Silent Problem

Almost all surgical procedures cause mild to severe postoperative pain and suffering. It is common for patients to tell us that no one prepared them for the amount of pain and discomfort they experienced after surgery. Pain is a mysterious and rarely discussed topic between patient and surgeon, yet it is one of the most feared aspects of the surgical experience. This silence reflects at least two attitudes. First, pain is an uncomfortable topic for both patient and surgeon and it is therefore avoided in order to minimize the patient's anxiety. Second, the surgeon is mainly focused on curing the patient's condition and may, therefore, consider pain an unavoidable and harmless consequence of surgery that simply has to be endured for a short time following the operation.

Although not all postoperative pain can or should be eliminated, there is now considerable scientific evidence that pain is not harmless. In fact, research shows that pain is not healthy and has profound physical and emotional consequences. As soon as the body experiences pain, long-lasting changes occur in the nervous system that make the nerves more sensitive to pain. Excessive postoperative pain may result in many potentially harmful physical and emotional complications which impair the healing and recovery process. These facts have prompted Dr. John C. Liebeskind, a member of the National Academy of Sciences, former president of the American Pain Society, and president-elect of the International Association for the Study of Pain, to state bluntly that *pain can kill*. His research shows that pain has a deleterious effect on the immune system which may interfere with healing (Liebeskind 1991).

There are, in fact, many potentially severe and even life-threatening complications that can result from excessive postoperative pain. Some of these are as follows:

- Pain may lead to shallow breathing and cough suppression in an attempt to "splint" or guard the injured area. This results in retained pulmonary secretions ("water in the lungs") that can cause pneumonia.

- Unrelieved pain may delay the return of gastric motility and bowel function following surgery.

- Pain may delay activities such as getting out of bed, moving, and exercising that are critically important for recovery. Excessive inactivity can increase the risk of inflammation in the veins which may cause dangerous blood clotting.

- Excessive pain may also result in increased need for pain medications which, when taken incorrectly, can have side effects that can impede recovery from surgery.

As well as the problems described above, excessive postoperative pain may cause emotional reactions such as stress, anxiety, and depression, which in turn, may create significant postoperative complications. The emotional suffering caused by pain not only reduces pain tolerance but, combined with the physical stress of surgery, causes the release of *stress hormones*. These stress hormones impair the immune function and promote the breakdown of body tissue, which results in poor recovery and healing. In addition, the more you suffer the easier it is to give up and withdraw from active participation in your recovery.

Since excessive pain results in slower recovery and healing times, longer postoperative hospital stays are inevitable. This increases the costs to both patient and insurance provider. Excessive postoperative pain also reduces the patient's satisfaction with the surgical experience even though the surgery may have been very successful in curing the problem. Untreated pain creates the greatest physical and emotional risk among patients who are young, older and frail patients with other illnesses such as heart or lung disease, or patients who are undergoing major surgical procedures such as open-heart surgery or organ transplants.

Government Guidelines for Pain Control

Recognition of the widespread inadequacy of postoperative pain management in hospitals throughout the United States prompted Congress, through the Agency for Health Care Policy and Research (AHCPR), to commission a panel of pain management experts to develop guidelines for the management of acute postoperative pain in adults and children.

In 1992, these experts who represent many health care specialties, including medicine, nursing, psychology, pharmacy, medical ethics, and patient consumers, published a revolutionary document entitled *Clinical Practice Guidelines for Acute Pain Management: Operative or Medical Procedures and Trauma.*

The AHCPR guidelines have four major goals:

1. To reduce the incidence and severity of postoperative or posttraumatic pain

2. To educate patients about the need to communicate unrelieved pain in order to receive prompt evaluation and effective treatment

3. To enhance patient comfort and satisfaction

4. To reduce postoperative complications and, in some cases, the length of hospital stays

The AHCPR guidelines are available free from the address listed in the References and Resources section.

Bad News and Good News

The bad news is that the problem of postsurgical pain is epidemic. Research indicates that over half of all persons undergoing surgery have inadequate pain relief! This is true even when patients are given routine intramuscular (IM) injections of powerful pain medications, such as narcotics, on an as-needed basis. (Agency for Health Care Policy and Research (AHCPR) 1992).

The good news is that the AHCPR guidelines reviewed important research showing that the great majority of postoperative pain is either preventable or controllable. See the sidebar entitled "Government Guidelines for Pain Control" (page 71). The AHCPR guidelines recommend a preventative approach which has as its cornerstone good patient-doctor communication. Your best weapon against pain is communication, and that communication needs to be clear and assertive. Become informed, ask questions, and explore your options. You need to break the silence and talk to your doctor about pain and pain control options. By doing so you will fight two major causes of unnecessary pain: the anxiety and depression that result from loss of control and fear of the unknown. The information in Chapter 12 will provide you with the necessary communication skills.

The remainder of this chapter provides you with twelve steps to establish a pain control plan and break the silence of pain. The steps show you how to discuss and plan a pain control strategy with your surgeon. Remember, you have a right to adequate pain relief and it is the ethical obligation of your surgical team to assist you with safe and effective pain management. Don't be shy, explore your pain control options and agree on a plan with your doctor and surgical team that makes sense to you. An open and frank discussion about your pain control options is a big step toward establishing a positive working relationship with your surgeon and surgical team.

Twelve Steps to Establish a Pain Control Plan

The following twelve steps will help you help yourself. Discuss each step with your surgeon and surgical team:

STEP 1: Ask your surgeon if the hospital has an established surgical pain control service.

Many hospitals have *surgical pain control services* that are responsible for postoperative pain management. If your surgeon operates in several hospitals, we strongly suggest choosing the one with a surgical pain control service. This is especially important if your specific surgery might result in significant postoperative pain and, of course, if there are no other *medical* reasons that would compel your surgeon to choose another hospital. Typically, those hospitals that have set a high priority on pain relief by establishing a surgical pain service provide the most effective pain management. To avoid confusion, it is important to have one individual or service in charge of your pain control. Ask your doctor the following questions and record the information on the appropriate lines:

Does the designated hospital have an established surgical pain service? If not, does the surgeon operate in a hospital that does and can my surgery be scheduled there?

_____

_____

_____

_____

If there is not an established surgical pain service, who will be in charge of managing my pain? Write down the name and phone number of this individual.

_____

_____

_____

_____

STEP 2: Talk to your doctor about pain control.

Prior to developing a pain control plan with your surgeon and surgical team it is important to talk to your doctors about the following:

- Pain control methods that have and have not worked well for you in the past

- Any concerns you may have about pain medication

- Any allergies you may have to medications (these should be recorded on your medical fact sheet)

- The medicines you take for other health problems (mixing some drugs with some pain medicines can cause problems—these are also recorded on your medical fact sheet)

STEP 3: Ask your surgeon and surgical team member what to expect.

In our experience we have observed most doctors and health care professionals have a tendency to minimize discussions about what you may feel following the surgery. It seems that they believe this silence will reduce your anxiety and distress. In reality, this silence actually may be harmful to you. As discussed previously, research has repeatedly found that most people who are provided with accurate *sensory information* show decreased postoperative pain, use less pain medication, and decrease their length of stay in the hospital following surgery. Sensory information describes how you will feel after surgery. Answers to the following questions will provide you with sensory information about your postoperative recovery.

Will there be much pain after surgery?

_____

_____

_____

_____

What will the pain feel like?

_____

_____

_____

_____

Where will the pain occur?

_____

_____

_____

_____

How long is the pain likely to last?

_____

_____

_____

_____

How long will it be before I can be active?

_____

_____

_____

_____

Will there be any side effects to the treatment (such as nausea)? How long will these last?

_____

_____

_____

_____

When you have satisfactory and detailed answers to these questions, there shouldn't be any major surprises regarding pain and discomfort or side effects following your surgery.

STEP 4: Discuss your pain medication options with your surgeon and surgical team.

There are many pain management options available to you. Some of these involve the use of pain medications and others do not. It is important to understand these options prior to your surgery. While there are many approaches to choose from, analgesic or pain medications are the mainstay of postoperative pain relief. Here are some choices of analgesic medications and options for medication delivery.

Options for Analgesic Medications

Nonsteroidal Anti-Inflammatory Drugs (NSAIDs). NSAIDs are the most commonly used medications to relieve mild to moderate pain. These medications also can be effective in reducing soreness, swelling, and inflammation. This class of medication includes acetaminophen, aspirin, ibuprofen, and other NSAIDs.

Benefits: There is no risk of addiction to NSAIDs. Depending on how much pain you have, these medicines can lessen or eliminate the need for stronger medications such as morphine and other narcotics.

Risks: Most NSAIDs interfere with blood clotting. They may cause nausea, stomach bleeding, or when used for long periods, kidney problems. For severe pain, a narcotic usually must be added.

Are You Afraid of Addiction to Pain Medicines?

Opioids are the mainstays of postoperative pain management. Opioids are the narcotic and narcotic-like medications routinely used for surgical pain control. Many people avoid or even refuse the use of narcotics because of fear of addiction. Also due to this fear, some patients do not take the pain medicine in adequate doses to give relief. In addressing these concerns it is important to distinguish between tolerance, dependence, and addiction.

Tolerance is a well-known pharmacologic property of all narcotics. It is a normal reaction in which the body gets used to the effect of the medication over time, sometimes requiring an increase in the dose.

Dependence occurs due to chemical events in the body. If the medicine is suddenly stopped, physical withdrawal might occur.

Addiction is the *psychological* craving for the medication even when it is not necessary for pain relief.

Tolerance and dependence are normal physical occurrences that are easily managed when pain medication is required for longer periods of time. The latest research on millions of postoperative patients has demonstrated that *addiction* to analgesics from legitimate pain control is virtually impossible. Narcotics are a safe and effective means of pain control. Don't worry!

Opioids: These are the narcotic and narcotic-like medications that are the most powerful pain medications currently available. The most commonly used medications for surgical pain include morphine and codeine, among others.

Benefits: These medicines are effective for severe pain, and they do not cause bleeding in the stomach or elsewhere. It is rare for a patient to become addicted as a result of taking opioids for postoperative pain.

Risks: Opioids may cause drowsiness, nausea, constipation, or itching, or may interfere with breathing or urination.

Local Anesthetics: Local anesthetics, similar to those used by your dentist to numb a tooth, may also be considered. These drugs may be given topically or by injection in the area of the surgical incision in order to numb that area and block the transmission of pain messages to the spinal cord. Local anesthetics also may be given through a small tube placed in your back, to block the nerves that transmit pain messages.

Benefits: Topical anesthetics are easy to apply and may be very effective for minor surgical procedures. Local anesthetics that are injected are effective for severe pain and have a rapid onset time. There is little or no risk of drowsiness, constipation, or breathing problems. Local anesthetics may reduce the need for opioid use.

Risks: Some people are allergic to topical anesthetic creams. When injections are used they may need to be repeated to maintain pain relief. An overdose of local anesthetic can have serious consequences. Average doses may cause some patients dizziness or weakness in their legs.

Options for Medication Delivery

In addition to the variety of medications available for pain relief, there are also many different ways in which many of them may be administered or *delivered.* Some delivery methods may be more effective than others, depending on your particular situation. The methods of medication delivery which have been adapted from the AHCPR guidelines are these:

Tablet or liquid. The most common medications are those given by mouth. These include aspirin, NSAIDs, and opioid medications such as codeine or morphine.

Benefits: Tablets and liquids cause less discomfort than injections into muscle or skin, and they can work just as well. They are inexpensive, simple to give, and easy to use at home. Since we all have some experience taking medications by mouth, oral delivery tends to be the safest method under most circumstances.

Risks: These medicines are not an option if nothing can be taken by mouth or if you are nauseated or vomiting. In such cases, sometimes these medicines can be administered rectally using a suppository. If you are using tablets, liquids, or suppositories, there may be a delay in pain relief because you must ask for the medicine and wait for it to be brought to you.

Injections into skin or muscle. Most pain medications and local anesthetics can be delivered by injection into the skin or muscle.

Benefits: Medicine given by injection into skin or muscle is effective even if you are nauseated or vomiting; such injections are simple to give and can provide fast relief.

Risks: The injection site is usually painful for a short time, especially if repeated injections are required. Medicines given by injection are more expensive than tablets or liquids. Pain relief may be delayed while you ask the nurse for medicine and wait for the shot to be prepared and administered.

Injections into a vein. Pain medicines are injected into a vein through a small tube, called an intravenous (IV) catheter. The tip of the tube stays in the vein.

Benefits: Medicines injected into a vein are fully absorbed and act very quickly. This method is especially effective for relief of brief episodes of intense pain. To relieve ongoing pain the IV catheter may be attached to a pump designed to deliver the medication at a constant infusion rate. The IV may also be equipped with a button that the patient can press to deliver more medicine when experiencing increased pain. This process is called Patient Controlled Analgesia or PCA. (See Step 5 for more information.) These various forms of IV delivery are excellent methods for managing severe postoperative pain that has been unresponsive to other routes of delivery.

Risks: Because a small tube must be inserted in a vein the possibility of infection must be closely monitored. Also, there are extra costs for pumps, supplies, and staff time.

Injections into the spine. In this method, narcotics or local anesthetics are given through a small tube (called an epidural or intrathecal catheter) inserted into the spine or the area surrounding your spine. Optimally the catheter is inserted prior to your surgery by an anesthesiologist and may be left in after surgery to facilitate pain control.

Benefits: Whether using morphine or a local anesthetic, this method is a very effective means of controlling severe pain either in discrete locations or over large areas of your body.

Risks: Staff must be specially trained to place a small tube in the back and to watch for problems that can appear hours after the medication is given. Infection is also a possibility with this method. Extra cost is involved for staff time, training, and supplies.

STEP 5: Talk to your doctor about the schedule for pain medicines in the hospital.

Some patients receive pain medication in the hospital only when their pain becomes severe enough for them to call the nurse. This is called p.r.n. (pro re nata) or as-needed scheduling. If the nursing staff is busy, has to prepare the medication, or does not have the specific medication available, as-needed schedules may result in delays and an increase of pain while you wait. The delays cause significant emotional distress for you and for your family who must sit passively by and watch you suffer. Also, these delays are a potential but avoidable source of conflict between the patient and the nursing staff. Giving medications on a p.r.n. or as-needed basis is considered to be relatively ineffective, especially if you have undergone major surgery.

Two major advances in the way pain medications are scheduled have resulted in significant improvements in postoperative control of pain. These are time-contingent scheduling and patient-controlled analgesia.

Time-Contingent Scheduling

Time-contingent scheduling requires giving the pain medication at set times whether or not the pain is severe. Instead of waiting until pain gets worse or "breaks through" the effect of the previous medication, you receive the medicine at set times during the day to keep the pain under control. For example, if you are likely to have pain requiring opioids for forty-eight hours following surgery, the surgeon may order morphine to be administered every four hours around the clock rather than on an as-needed basis. Thus, *time* determines when you get the medication rather than the severity of the pain. By giving medications in this time-contingent manner, the physician can adjust the doses to establish a constant level of pain medication in the blood.

Time-contingent dosing avoids the "peaks and valleys" of pain that characterize as-needed dosing. In as-needed dosing, you may feel great for a short time after you are given the medication. But as the medication wears off you watch the clock until increasing pain again forces you to request the next dose. Patients often tell us that as-needed dosing make them feel like they are on a roller-coaster ride with their pain.

Time-contingent scheduling is one of the most important advances in the effective use of pain medications. It virtually eliminates the roller-coaster aspects of as-needed scheduling. Later in your postoperative recovery, it may be acceptable to change to as-needed scheduling as healing renders your pain more manageable.

Patient-Controlled Analgesia (PCA)

The second major advancement in pain medication scheduling and delivery is called Patient-Controlled Analgesia or PCA. A small catheter or tube placed in the vein is connected to a pump that delivers predetermined amounts of pain medication when you push a button. PCA puts you in charge of your pain management by allowing you to control when the pain medicine is delivered. When you begin to feel pain, you press a button to inject the medicine through the intravenous (IV) tube in your vein. Built-in safety measures prevent you from giving yourself too much medication. The results are immediate because you control the dose and do not have to wait for the nursing staff to respond to your requests for medications.

PCA is the preferred method of pain control following most major surgeries. Many research studies have found that patients using PCA are much more comfortable, use less pain medication overall, can be discharged from the hospital earlier, and are generally more satisfied with their care. You should discuss this remarkable option with your surgeon. However, not all hospitals have PCA technology available.

STEP 6: Talk to your surgeon about your anesthesia options.

The basic purpose of anesthesia is to eliminate pain and distress so that you may safely undergo a surgical procedure. Many options have been made available in anesthesia. Depending on the nature of your surgery you may choose to avoid being "put under" or rendered unconscious with a general anesthetic, since this procedure carries with it certain risks. The range of choices for anesthesia may seem bewildering, so it is very important to review the options carefully with your surgeon and anesthesiologist. We highly recommend meeting with your anesthesiologist before your scheduled surgery. Choose the mode of anesthesia that is least risky and invasive but will safely and adequately control pain.

Anesthesia is generally local, regional, or general.

Local Anesthesia

Local anesthesia is the injection of anesthetic medication around the site of the surgical incision or somewhere along a major nerve which serves the area. Topical sprays or drops into the throat, eyes, and mouth can be effective for minor surgical procedures. Anesthetic creams are also effective for minor surgical procedures, especially in children. These methods temporarily numb the area of the surgery while leaving the rest of the body unaffected. This can be the safest, least invasive, and most effective means of controlling pain for many surgical procedures. With local anesthesia you may be able to avoid a general anesthetic. In some cases, your doctor may use a sedative in combination with the local anesthetic to calm you and reduce your stress.

Regional Anesthesia

In regional anesthesia, a local anesthetic medication is injected into the spine or into the area adjacent to your spine, producing profound numbness over large areas of your body. For example, in spinal and epidural blocks, a small plastic tube or catheter is placed in the space surrounding your spine, through which a local anesthetic can be continuously delivered. If appropriate, delivery of the anesthetic through the catheter can continue even after the surgery is over. In some instances, morphine can be delivered through the same catheter, producing excellent pain relief with few side effects.

Regional anesthesia works particularly well for chest surgery or for operations on the lower parts of your body such as hip and knee replacements or prostate surgery. It is the most widely used method for controlling the pain of childbirth, especially if a Caesarean section is performed, allowing the mother to be conscious during the delivery. It may also be a better choice than other anesthesia options for patients with multiple or complicated medical problems. Research has demonstrated that in appropriate cases spinal anesthesia can reduce postoperative complications and pain, as well as hasten recovery. Regional anesthesia may enable you to avoid a general anesthetic during surgery and to remain conscious during a surgical procedure so that you can tell your surgical team if anything feels uncomfortable. Of course your anesthesiologist can also administer sedative medications to keep you calm.

General Anesthesia

In general anesthesia you are rendered unconscious by a combination of IV drugs (e.g., sodium thiopentone), muscle relaxants (e.g., curare), and anesthetic gases (e.g., isoflurane and halothane mixed with oxygen). These drugs may slow or depress important physiological functions such as breathing and heart rate. Therefore, close monitoring by the anesthesiologist is absolutely necessary. The placement of an endotracheal tube (in the throat) may also be required to control breathing.

General anesthesia is the most widely used type of anesthesia for major surgeries. It is the method of choice for patients who prefer to be totally "asleep" and unaware during their surgical experience. But general anesthesia is not without risks. Sometimes patients react to the general anesthetics after the surgery by feeling dizzy or nauseous or "spaced-out." Although general anesthesia is extremely safe, you should discuss with your surgeon and anesthesiologist the risks and benefits of the various options for anesthesia.

STEP 7: Talk to your surgeon about preemptive analgesia.

Preemptive analgesia, potentially a very effective technique, has been the subject of much recent research. Discuss this procedure with your surgeon and anesthesiologist. Preemptive analgesia is based on the previously discussed research showing that pain messages from tissue damage, such as that which occurs during surgery, may cause lasting changes in the nervous system that can make you *hypersensitive* to pain. The object of preemptive analgesia is to *prevent* or *preempt* pain messages from reaching the spinal cord, so that these lasting changes will not occur. Thus, preemptive analgesia normally requires taking action *before* the surgery is performed. This may be done by:

- Injecting or infiltrating local anesthetics into the tissue or area of the surgery

- Injecting local anesthetics around the nerves responsible for transmitting the pain message to the spinal cord

- Injecting the spine with a local anesthetic in order to block nerve impulses

- Giving the patient opioid medications, nonsteroidal anti-inflammatory drugs (NSAIDs), or other pain-relieving medications before the surgery

In some cases these preemptive procedures are completed during the actual surgery. The underlying principle is that the treatment is done in advance of the pain rather than in reaction to it. The research, which is promising, has shown that patients given preemptive analgesia usually have less postoperative pain and require less postoperative pain medication. Keep in mind that preemptive analgesia is a relatively new technique and is not yet widely used. Discuss this option with your surgeon and anesthesiologist, especially if you are experiencing pain prior to your surgery. Evidence suggests that preemptive analgesia can keep presurgical pain, especially nerve-related or neuropathic pain, from becoming more severe during surgery (Woolf and Chong 1993).

STEP 8: Be sure to discuss with your doctors the option of pain control without medication.

Although the main focus of this chapter has been on *medications* for the control of postoperative pain, there are several *nonmedication* techniques that can be very effective. Most pain is best treated through a combination of these methods. The nonmedication approaches listed below are readily available, easy to use, inexpensive, and entail little risk. Explore these options with your surgeon and surgical team. If they are available to you, find out in advance how to arrange for them. Discuss the following nonmedication pain management techniques with your surgeon:

- *Patient Education*: You should be informed about all aspects of your surgery. The questionnaires in Chapter 3 can help you get adequate information. If you are having major surgery, make sure you have been instructed about proper physiological coping techniques such as coughing, deep breathing, turning, and ambulation (walking). Patients given such instruction prior to surgery report that they experience less pain, require fewer pain medications, and have shorter hospital stays. Find out if your hospital has a presurgical education class. If it doesn't, you may want to meet with a member of the nursing team who can instruct you.

- *Cognitive-Behavioral and Relaxation Techniques*: There is extensive scientific evidence that relaxation, imagery, music, and cognitive-behavioral techniques, which are discussed later in this book, are extremely effective in reducing pain and suffering. These techniques are easy to learn and have no negative consequences.

- *Heat and Cold*: Applying heat and cold may reduce pain sensitivity, reduce muscle spasms, and decrease congestion in an injured area (for example, the site of surgery). The initial application of cold decreases tissue injury response, and later, heat can promote the clearance of tissue toxins and accumulated fluids.

- *Massage and Exercise*: Massage and exercise are used to stretch and regain muscle and tendon length and expand the range of motion. In spinal surgeries and surgeries of the extremities (shoulders, arms, and legs) these techniques are especially important.

- *Immobilization*:   Immobilization devices such as casts and braces are typically used after musculoskeletal surgeries to provide rest and maintain the alignment necessary for proper healing.

- *Transcutaneous Electrical Nerve Stimulation (TENS)*: TENS is a technique for pain control and healing in which adhesive pads containing electrodes are placed in specific pain locations following surgery or injury. The electrodes are connected by thin wires to a pocket-sized, battery-operated stimulator that produces an adjustable electric current. The electric current, which produces a tingling sensation, is thought to decrease pain by raising the pain threshold of the nerves in the spinal cord that respond to injury. TENS may also promote healing by reducing inflammation and increasing mobilization following surgery. TENS has been successfully used with thousands of patents and is particularly helpful after abdominal, spinal, and chest surgeries.

When used appropriately, these techniques are safe and effective. They will not mask potential problems that might arise following surgery, and they have no significant side effects. We highly recommend that, when indicated, they should be fully integrated into any postoperative pain management plan.

STEP 9: *The key to effective pain management is to stay ahead of your pain.*

The most important thing to remember for effective pain management is to *stay ahead of your pain* by taking pain medications and using nonmedication techniques when the pain first begins or even before it starts. Once the pain escalates and gets out of hand it is very difficult to regain control of it. Stay ahead of your pain by doing the following:

- Take action as soon as the pain starts to increase by immediately using your pain medications and nonpharmacological techniques (e.g., ice, TENS, relaxation).

- If you know that certain activities such as stretching, walking, coughing, or breathing exercises will increase your pain, then take your pain medications and use your nonmedication approaches first, before engaging in the painful activity.

- When engaging in activities that will increase pain, stay ahead of your pain by carefully pacing yourself. Do not engage in an activity to the point that pain or fatigue forces you to stop. Rather, stop well before pain or fatigue overtake you and rest for a short time. Then resume the activity for a short period, again followed by a short rest. Repeat this sequence until the activity is complete. In this way, by staying ahead of the pain and deciding when to stop, you have gained both a physical and psychological advantage over your pain. In the management of postoperative pain, the idea of "no pain, no gain" is wrong and harmful.

STEP 10: *Help the doctors and nurses "measure" your pain.*

No matter which pain medications or delivery methods are used to control your post-operative pain, your nurses and doctors will ask you how the pain medicine is working. They will change the medicine, dose, or scheduling if you are having excessive pain. Since the medication is adjusted in response to your own evaluation of your pain, you must be accurate and honest in your reporting. You need to agree with your doctors and nurses on a method of reporting your pain. If your hospital has an established acute pain service, your pain may be measured in a standardized way.

A numerical rating scale may be the easiest to use.

- **Numerical Rating Scale:** In this method you rate your pain on a scale of 0 (*No Pain*) to 10 (*Most Intense Pain Imaginable*). A rating of 10 may not necessarily mean your worst pain. Under some circumstances, your pain may exceed any that you have previously experienced. Therefore, a rating of 10 may not mean your worst possible pain, but the worst pain you can *ever* imagine having.

- **Visual Analog Scale (VAS):** Another scale that is frequently used is the VAS. The VAS is a horizontal straight line, usually 10 cm in length. The left end represents *No Pain* and the right end the *Most Intense Pain Imaginable*. There are many forms of the VAS. The example shown has numerical and descriptive features. You are asked to mark the line to indicate the intensity of your pain.

```
|---|---|---|---|---|---|---|---|---|---|
```

| 0 | 1 | 2 | 3 | 4 | 5 | 6 | 7 | 8 | 9 | 10 |

No Pain   Moderate Pain   Most Intense Pain Imaginable

You may determine with your doctor and surgeon a pain control goal in which your pain will not be allowed to exceed a specified level such as 3 out of 10, for example. A pain level in excess of this would then prompt an adjustment in your medication. Using a number to report your pain helps the doctors and nurses to evaluate how well your treatment is working and to decide if any changes need to be made.

Rating your pain and frequently recording your pain levels can also help with effective pain control. It is useful to rate and record pain levels when you wake up in the morning, at midday, early evening, and just before you go to sleep at night. Record any comments or notes about your pain that you want the surgical team to know. For example:

Time	Pain (0–10)	Notes
8 AM	4	Aching has increased
12 PM	2	
4 PM	5	Walking, pain sharp
8 PM	1	No nausea
2 AM	5	A brief, sharp pain woke me up

STEP 11: *Tell your doctor or nurse about any persistent pain.*

Don't worry about being a bother when it comes to reporting symptoms, including pain, to your doctors and nurses. Your medical team want and need to know about your pain. Any change, especially in severity or quality (for example, pain that was dull has become sharp and shooting) may be a sign of problems that require immediate attention.

STEP 12: *Ask your doctor how your pain will be controlled after you are discharged from the hospital.*

Patients who are experiencing pain at the time of discharge from the hospital are generally given oral medications to take with them. These are usually to be taken on a strict time-contingent schedule, as discussed in Step 5. For example, you may be prescribed ibuprofen (Motrin; Nuprin), hydrocodone (Vicodin; Lorcet) or oxycodone (Percocet) to be taken every four or six hours, depending on the severity of your pain and the degree of relief you achieve. As you feel better, the amount of medication should be gradually reduced until you need only one or two doses a day as needed. As your pain subsides, you may be told to switch to over-the-counter pain medicines. If after your discharge you have significant pain and are taking frequent doses of narcotic medications, it is best to remain in contact with your surgeon or pain medicine physician every one or two weeks, then less frequently as your pain subsides. *Note that if your are experiencing pain before your surgery the same suggestions apply. It is equally important to stabilize and monitor your pain medications and pain before surgery—that is, strict time-contingent scheduling of pain medications and frequent follow-up visits to your doctor. If you take too much pain medication before your surgery this may cause side effects or put you at risk for inadequate pain control following your surgery.*

As a general guiding principle, remember to stay ahead of your pain by not waiting too long to take the medications and by pacing your activities. You will also want to use the nonpharmacological techniques discussed in Step 8. We have found that relaxation techniques are especially effective for pain control.

PART III

Training for Healthy Self-Talk

Part III helps you to prepare your *mind* for surgery. In Chapter 5 we present the concept of negative thoughts and self-talk as critical in their affect on your physical and emotional response to surgery. In this chapter you learn to identify your conscious and unconscious negative thoughts and self-talk using a journal. Chapter 6 shows how to identify styles of negative self-talk and presents you with techniques for challenging them and ways to replace negative self-talk with coping self-talk and positive affirmations.

After reading Part III you will understand the following.

1. The role of thoughts and self-talk on your emotional state and surgical experience

2. How to identify negative thoughts and self-talk

3. How to categorize and appraise negative thoughts and self-talk

4. How to stop negative thoughts and replace them with coping self-talk and positive affirmations

5

Unconscious Thoughts and Self-Talk

There is nothing either good or bad, but thinking makes it so.

—William Shakespeare, *Hamlet*

Surgery causes mental and physical stress. To control this stress you must understand what is occurring both in your mind and body. Your mind generates thoughts which, in turn, affect your emotions, your body, your response to surgery, and your recovery.

To illustrate how thoughts can cause different responses to the same situation, consider the following example:

> Sue absolutely loves to travel by airplane. She views the airplane trip as an opportunity to take a break from her busy schedule. It is a time when she can relax and enjoy herself, and when no demands can be made on her by others. During the flight her body is relaxed and she may nap, read a book, or watch a movie. She truly feels that flying is a nice break from the stress of her everyday responsibilities.
>
> Cheryl, on the other hand, dreads airplane trips. She hates packing for the trip, getting to the airport, and waiting for the flight to take off. She finds being cooped up in the plane for several hours very stressful, and she can hardly wait for the trip to end. She sees it as a waste of time during which she gets nothing productive accomplished. Her physical reactions include increased heart rate, muscle tension, and stomach upset.

Why do Sue and Cheryl have such very different emotional and physical reactions to the same situation? The differences are the result of their thoughts. Sue's thinking includes such ideas as, "I can sit and relax for a few hours," "No one can bother me," and "Maybe I will meet some nice people." Cheryl's thoughts include, "I can't stand to fly and I never will," "I hate being packed in like a sardine," and "Flying is a total waste of time."

Self-Talk

We all constantly judge and interpret the world around us. These thoughts and judgments, both conscious and unconscious, have been termed "self-talk" because they are like dialogues with ourselves. Often, an internal dialogue is so quick and automatic that we do not notice its exact content. Rather, we experience only the emotional and physical reactions caused by the self-talk.

Self-talk, and its subsequent emotions, can have a healthy, positive effect or an unhealthy, negative effect. In the psychological process of preparing for surgery and enhancing your outcome, your state of mind is extremely important. The connection between thoughts, emotions, and physical states is illustrated further in the following examples. In each situation you can see that there are two possible sets of self-talk scenarios that can lead to very different emotional and physical responses.

Situation A

Your date is late for dinner after telling you he (or she) would meet you at a specific time and place.

Self-Talk

- I knew he'd been acting funny lately, I bet there's a problem.

- He's never late—maybe he didn't really want to meet me.

- I'm not interesting enough for him to want to be with me.

- I should have seen it coming—he's going to break up with me.

- He's not going to show up at all.

- Our relationship is over. I'll never have a relationship that works.

Emotional Response

- Anger

- Depression

- Frustration

- Helplessness

Physical Response

- Heart rate increase

- Breathing rate increase

- Muscle tension

Behavioral Response

- Have more to drink than you usually do

- Have a cigarette even though you don't smoke

- Leave the restaurant after waiting 15 minutes

Alternative Self-Talk

- He's very prompt—something must have happened to delay him.

- The traffic is bad—maybe he's stuck on the freeway.

- He would call if he could get to a phone.

Alternative Emotional Response

- Mild distress or concern

Alternative Physical Response

- No change from usual state or slight physical arousal related to being concerned

Alternative Behavioral Response

- Wait at the restaurant a reasonable amount of time until he arrives

- Try and call him or a friend/business colleague

Situation B

You are suffering from chronic back and neck pain which is primarily muscular in nature. No serious condition has been identified and the doctors have encouraged you to go on with your normal life.

Self-Talk

- There is something seriously wrong with my spine.

- My spine is weak and fragile.

- My pain is going to get worse and worse.

- I can't cope with this pain.

- I'll never get better.

- I'll always have pain.

- I should be better by now.

- My back pain is all "their" fault.

- Nobody really understands my pain.

- If I move the wrong way, I'll cripple myself.

Emotional Response

- Hopelessness

- Helplessness

- Anxiety and fear

- Depression

- Anger

Physical Response

- A stress response including muscle tension, increase in heart rate, and rapid breathing.

Behavioral Response

- Staying in bed

- Social isolation

- Physical inactivity

- Absence from work

- Overuse of pain medicines

- Groaning, moaning, and grimacing

- Slow, robot-like movements

Alternative Self-Talk

- My spine is strong.

- It is good for me to move and be active.

- There are ways for me to distract myself from the pain.

- I can cope with this pain until it subsides.

- I'm trying to get better.

- There are things I can do to enjoy life.

Alternative Emotional Response

- A decrease in negative, unpleasant emotions and a greater sense of control

Alternative Physical Response

- A decrease in the overall physical stress response

Alternative Behavioral Response

- Getting up and out of bed

- Deciding to call a friend to go out

- Taking a short walk

- Doing volunteer work or some other purposeful activity

- Moving as smoothly and fluidly as possible

These examples show that your thinking impacts your emotions, physical state, and behavior. Some self-talk is conscious (or in the person's awareness) and some of it is unconscious (not in the person's awareness). Self-talk can affect you whether you are aware of it or not.

As these examples illustrate, self-talk can be either positive (healthy) or negative (unhealthy). Depending on many factors, individuals seem to be more likely to engage in one or the other. Those prone to more positive self-talk on a regular basis are called optimists while those who generally engage in negative self-talk are called pessimists.

This chapter will help you to identify the negative self-talk that can cause problems related to your surgical experience and recovery. For example, the following statements represent unhealthy or negative self-talk:

- I will never be able to stand the surgery.

- There will be too much pain to endure.

- The hospital is a very scary place.

- The surgery will not be successful.

- I just can't tell the doctor about my concerns.

If you are having thoughts like these, your emotional state is likely to be anxious and depressed. In addition, your physical responses might include a slower rate of healing and a higher susceptibility to infection (decreased immune function).

Examples of healthy unconscious thoughts or self-talk might include such beliefs as the following:

- I am choosing to have this surgery for its positive outcome, which will be . . .

- I can take control of my situation in the following ways . . .

- I can cope with the pain and discomfort by . . .

- I am looking forward to having the surgery completed and getting on with my recovery.

Are You an Optimist or a Pessimist?

Do you tend to agree or disagree with the following statements? Try not to respond with what you think people *should* say or what sounds correct, but how you really view your life.

1. I usually expect the best in uncertain times.
2. If something can go wrong for me, it will.
3. I always look at the bright side of things.
4. I hardly ever expect things to go my way.
5. I am always optimistic about my future.
6. Things never work out the way I want them to.
7. I am a believer in the idea that "every cloud has a silver lining."
8. I rarely count on good things happening to me.

If you tended to agree with the odd-numbered items (1,3,5,7) and disagree with the even-numbered items (2,4,6,8), then you are more of an optimist. If you tended to agree with the even-numbered items and disagree with the odd-numbered items, then you are more of a pessimist.

If your thoughts about surgery follow this healthy pattern, then your emotional and physical states are likely to be much more positive.

Unhealthy self-talk tends to have the following characteristics:

- It takes the form of specific, discrete messages that often are expressed in shorthand

- You find it highly believable no matter how unhealthy or irrational it is

- It is experienced as highly spontaneous and difficult to "turn off"

- It is often expressed in terms of *should, ought, never, always,* and *must*

- Self-talk is unique to you as an individual.

Becoming Aware of Negative Self-Talk

Learning to be aware of your unhealthy self-talk is the first step in changing it. At first, the nature of your self-talk may not be readily apparent to you, even though it is influencing your emotions and your body's health. Self-talk can be difficult to "catch" because it occurs so quickly. It is like watching a movie running at regular speed and trying to see one single frame at a time. It is simply not possible unless you change the movie speed to slow motion or freeze-frame. Then you can analyze the frame-by-frame sequences that make up the entire movie.

Similarly, there are ways to slow down and identify your self-talk: Use unpleasant emotions as a guide; watch for the tell-tale characteristics of unhealthy self-talk; and elaborate the shorthand messages completely.

Use Unpleasant Emotions as a Guide

Unhealthy self-talk can be identified by the negative emotions and/or physical reactions that it produces. Therefore, when you experience emotions such as depression, anger, anxiety, or fear, you can try to recreate the self-talk that preceded that emotion. For example, if you feel anxious about getting a diagnostic test, your self-talk might include statements like, "The test will be so painful I won't be able to handle it," "The test won't go well, they never do," and "They are going to find something awful."

Watch for the Signs of Unhealthy Self-Talk

Unhealthy self-talk often has specific characteristics that will be discussed more fully in Chapter 6. One such characteristic is the "should" statement, such as, "I *should* be doing better" or "I *should* have done this or that." Examples of other styles of unhealthy self-talk include thinking in all-or-nothing terms, exaggerating the negatives, and filtering out positive thoughts.

Elaborate the Shorthand Messages Completely

It can be very helpful to elaborate on the abbreviated shorthand message that is first identified as unhealthy self-talk. As an example, your initial analysis might be that you are anxious and depressed because you "feel sick." With some consideration and elaboration, you might discover an entire chain of unhealthy self-talk messages such as "I feel sick," and "There is nothing I can do about it," "I will always feel this way," "I should be feeling better," and, "There is nothing I can do to improve my situation."

How to Keep a Self-Talk Journal

You can practice identifying your unhealthy or negative self-talk by keeping a journal. When you experience an unpleasant emotion, write it down and then try to flush out as many unhealthy self-talk statements as possible that might add to that emotion. These statements might be related to your surgery, medical condition, family relationships, or any other part of your life.

To determine what may prompt your unhealthy self-talk, review your results on the questionnaires in Chapter 2 regarding depression, anxiety, anger, and hospital stress. The areas in which you scored above average may be those in which negative self-talk is likely to occur. Here are some examples of unhealthy self-talk in those areas.

Depression

- Nothing I do will help my situation.

- No matter what I do, I have no control.

- When I feel bad, there is nothing I can do about it.

- I feel worthless.

- Nobody cares about me.

- The future looks awful.

- I am sure this surgery will not work.

- I am useless.

Anxiety

- What if the surgery doesn't work?

- I can't handle being in the hospital.

- What if the pain is too great?

- I can't stand being away from home.

- All this medical information is too confusing.

- What if the doctors or nurses make a mistake?

Anger

- Everyone is treating me badly.

- My work is to blame for this injury.

- I don't deserve this medical problem.

- I'd be doing better if my family were supportive.

- It's always "Them against me."

- I'd be better off if my doctors paid more attention.

Hospital Stress

- Medical "stuff" always scares me.

- Doctors are always . . .

- People who go into the hospital don't come out.

- It will be embarrassing.

The following example may help you with your own journal.

Mike was very concerned about the major reconstructive dental surgery he needed. His worries concerned such broad areas as the surgery itself, his recovery, his time off work, and his financial burden, especially because he had no dental insurance. He had avoided going to the dentist even for minor check-ups, and now he was blaming himself excessively for needing the surgery. As the surgery date drew nearer he felt more irritable, depressed, angry, and anxious. He started the following self-talk journal:

Situation	Emotion	Unhealthy Self-Talk
Pain and bleeding in mouth	Depression	Why did this happen to me? I always have bad luck. This will never get better. My mouth is an awful mess.
Scheduling the surgery	Anxiety	I can't stand dental work. The sounds of the dentist's tools are unbearable. They won't be able to control the pain. What if the surgery doesn't work?
Talking with employer	Fear	I'm going to lose my job. Everyone is thinking, "Why didn't he take care of his teeth?"
Talking with doctor's office about payment	Anger	I should not have let this happen. These bills will ruin me. I'll never be able to pay this off.

Your Self-Talk Journal

Complete the following self-talk journal. Record your unhealthy self-talk whenever you experience an unpleasant emotional state or when you feel increased physical tension. First, record your situation when the feeling occurs. In some cases, you will not actually be in that situation but simply thinking about it (for instance, the stress of going to a doctor's office). Second, record all of the emotional responses you can, such as depression or anxiety. Last, write down all of the negative self-talk statements you can think of that might be related to your unpleasant emotions. Initially you may find that this last column is the most challenging. Do not become discouraged. As you use the journal, your patterns of negative, unhealthy self-talk will emerge. We will use this information in the following chapter.

Self Talk Journal

Situation	Emotion	Unhealthy Self-Talk

6

Retraining Your Self-Talk
and Developing the Power of
Healthy Thinking

If you have completed the Self-Talk Journal over several days, you will have developed some fertile material to help analyze your thoughts related to your surgery. This chapter discusses the various styles of negative self-talk, techniques for challenging these messages, and ways to develop affirmations to help you cope successfully with stress.

Styles of Negative Self-Talk

Researchers have identified specific styles of negative self-talk that lead to unpleasant emotions and stressful physical responses. These styles apply to any stressful situation, including surgery and postoperative recovery. These styles are summarized as follows:

Catastrophizing

This type of negative thinking is characterized by imagining the worst possible scenario and then acting as if that will actually happen. It may often include a series of "what ifs" such as:

- What if I never get better?

- What if I get worse?

- What if I can't help myself?

In catastrophic thinking, dire predictions are based on pessimistic beliefs rather than facts.

Filtering

In this thinking style you focus only on the negative aspects of a situation to the exclusion of any positive elements or options. This type of negative self-talk is also termed "tunnel vision" because it causes you to look only at one element of a situation to the exclusion of everything else. This style commonly includes searching for evidence of "how bad things really are" and discounting any positive or coping focus. Examples include the following kinds of statements:

- There is nothing that will help my situation.

- This situation is awful.

- Everything in my life is rotten due to this medical problem.

- Nobody really cares about me.

- I can't stand it.

- The doctors have nothing to offer.

- I've tried everything and nothing has helped at all.

This style of negative thinking is often characterized by discounting and "yes-butting." No matter what positive option or coping method is suggested, you discount it with a "yes-but." For instance, you require a surgical procedure that will limit certain activities while also improving your overall health and quality of life. When this is discussed as being very positive overall, you may retort, *"Yes, but* I will have these limitations." This type of thinking fosters helplessness, hopelessness, and depression.

Black-and-White Thinking

In this type of thinking, also termed "all-or-nothing" thinking, there is no middle ground nor any shades of gray. People and things are either good or bad. Events and situations are either great or horrible. Examples of this type of thinking are as follows:

- I'm either cured or I'm not.

- I either have pain or I don't.

- The treatment either works or it doesn't.

- This doctor is either good or bad.

- My family is supportive or they're not.

Black-and-white thinking undermines any small steps toward improvement, severely limits your options, and filters out any positive aspects of your situation.

Overgeneralization

In this process, an aspect of one situation is applied to all other situations, or a reaction to one situation is extended inappropriately to other situations. For instance:

- With this pain I'll never be able to have any fun.

- When I'm in pain nobody wants to be around me.

- My wife told me to try and do something about the pain. She must be ready to leave the marriage.

- I will always be sad and in pain.

- I will never be able to get beyond this awful medical problem.

This form of negative self-talk takes the substance of one incident and applies it to many other situations, resulting in an incorrect, overgeneralized conclusion. Overgeneralization is often indicated by such key words as *all, every, none, never, always, everybody,* and *nobody.*

Mind Reading

This negative self-talk "trap" involves making unsubstantiated assumptions about what other people are thinking, then acting on these often erroneous assumptions without verifying them. Examples of this might include the following:

- I know my wife thinks I'm less of a man because of my condition.

- I know my husband thinks I'm exaggerating.

- My doctor doesn't really think I'll get better, even though she tells me I will.

- They're not telling me everything about my problem.

If you accept these assumptions as facts, then your behavior will follow accordingly, and you are likely to create a self-fulfilling prophecy. For example, your spouse might ask, "How do you feel today?" Instead of taking his or her comment at face value, you believe he or she really means "Are you still letting that problem bother you?" So you respond, "How do you think I feel today? The same as always, that's how!" You can easily guess how this scenario might end.

Shoulds

"Should" statements are key elements in negative self-talk. In this style of negative self-talk, you operate from a list of inflexible and unrealistic rules about how you and other people *should* act or how situations *should* unfold. Examples of such thinking include:

- I should be getting better.

- I should never have allowed this to happen.

- I should have known not to have that procedure.

- My employer should have protected me.

- I should be tougher.

- My family should be more helpful.

"Should" thinking includes terms like *should, ought,* and *must.* "Should" thinking is very judgmental and often involves measuring your performance against some irrational perfect standard. This may make you feel worthless, useless, and inadequate. When directed at others, it may make you feel angry and resentful in those relationships.

Blaming

In blaming, you make something or someone else responsible for a problem or situation. You may feel some comfort in attaching responsibility for your suffering to someone else. Unfortunately, blaming can often cause you to avoid taking responsibility for your own choices and your opportunities for improvement. Very often this type of negative thinking arises in cases of industrial injuries, automobile accidents, or other similar traumas. Examples include the following:

- My boss is to blame for my injury.

- They should have mopped up that water I slipped on. It's all their fault.

- That guy who rear-ended me is responsible for for everything bad in my life.

Blaming as a form of negative self-talk can be focused either externally or internally. Internally focused blaming (self-blame) takes the form of, "It's all my fault." Self-blame is often an excuse for not taking responsibility and can lead to depression, hopelessness, and helplessness. Blaming can be very destructive. It keeps you from focusing on how to get better by diverting your attention on who or what is to blame.

Analyzing Your Self-Talk Style

As you consider these styles of negative self-talk, you may identify those patterns that you habitually use, and others that you rarely use. Although this book focuses on issues related to surgery, you may find that these thinking styles affect many other aspects of your life.

It is important to familiarize yourself with your styles of unhealthy negative self-talk. At this point, review your Self-Talk Journal and try to label the types of unhealthy self-talk recorded there. The next sections describe how to change your negative self-talk by challenging it and replacing it with *coping thoughts.*

Changing Your Self-Talk

There are simple, powerful, well-proven methods for changing negative self-talk. *It is essential to identify the negative self-talk as it occurs.* Try to catch yourself engaging in negative self-talk, first by noticing and identifying any unpleasant emotion or physical state and then by recording it in your journal.

Changing negative self-talk involves using three simple steps—thought stopping, challenging, and reframing. This can be easily remembered by these words—*stop, challenge,* and *reframe.*

Thought Stopping

Thought stopping is putting an abrupt halt to the cascade of negative self-talk messages as soon as you become aware of them. The moment you notice an unpleasant emotion, physical stress response, or actual negative self-talk, tell yourself to STOP. To make a more powerful impact, you might need to say it out loud. Some people even find it useful to visualize a stop sign.

Once you have stopped the flow of negative self-talk, you need to refocus your mind quickly on other types of thoughts called *coping* thoughts. Examples of coping thoughts follow:

- There's nothing to worry about.

- I can handle this situation.

- I'm going to be all right.

- I'll be through all of this soon.

- I have resources and people to help me.

- I can focus on positive thoughts.

- I'm doing the best I can.

- I can breathe deeply and relax.

- I can focus on the positive aspects of the operation.

- I feel peaceful.

In the space below, list other coping thoughts that relate to your specific situation and needs. Add to this list whenever you think of more coping thoughts. You might also find it useful to write these coping thoughts on an index card to keep with you, especially in the hospital and during your recovery from surgery. Reviewing these thoughts regularly, even when you are not stressed, is a good way to train yourself to use them more spontaneously.

_____

_____

_____

Challenging Negative Self-Talk

With these techniques you will *challenge* the reality and accuracy of your negative self-talk messages. Write down and rehearse positive, healthy self-talk messages that directly challenge your negative self-talk. Ask yourself the following questions to help challenge your negative self-talk:

- What is the evidence for that conclusion?

- Is this statement always true?

- What is the evidence for that conclusion being false?

- Among all possibilities, is this belief the healthiest one to adopt?

- Am I looking at the entire picture?

- Am I being fully objective?

Subjecting your self-talk to these questions helps you to distinguish between negative and positive messages. Develop positive messages keeping in mind the reality of your situation. If your messages are so positive as to be unbelievable, they will not be beneficial.

Thought Reframing

After identifying and challenging your negative self-talk, it is important to reframe it by substituting positive, realistic, or coping self-talk. Dr. Edmund Bourne (1995) developed the following rules to help write positive coping self-talk statements.

Avoid negatives. When writing your *positive* coping statement, avoid using *negatives*. For instance, instead of saying, "I can't be nervous about going to the hospital," tell yourself, "I will be confident and calm about going to the hospital." A negative statement can cause anxiety in and of itself and will defeat the purpose of the coping thought.

Keep coping thoughts in the present tense. Negative self-talk occurs spontaneously and affects you immediately. Challenge it with coping thoughts cast in the present tense. Instead of saying, "I will be happy when this surgery is over," tell yourself, "I am happy about . . . right now." Try beginning your self-statements with, "I am learning to . . ." and "I can. . . ."

Keep coping thoughts in the first person. Whenever possible it is helpful to formulate your thoughts in the first person. You can do this by beginning your coping thoughts with "I" or by being sure that "I" occurs somewhere in the sentence.

Make your coping thoughts believable. Coping thoughts should be based in reality. This will ensure that you have some belief in your coping self-talk. As you practice positive self-talk, it will become more and more believable to you. Don't make your coping thoughts too broadly positive or unrealistic, or you may discount them as untrue. For instance, the coping thought "I can't wait to have surgery. I'm sure I will completely enjoy the entire experience," is extremely unrealistic and unbelievable. Rather, the thought, "I will be able make the surgery experience as positive as possible and I will look forward to beginning my recovery" is much more tenable.

Examples of positive self-talk that challenges each of the negative styles follow:

Catastrophizing

When catastrophizing, remind yourself that no one can predict the future. Therefore, it is in your best interest to predict a realistic or positive outcome rather than a catastrophic one. Believing that things will turn out well is the best course of action. When you find yourself catastrophizing, remember the following statements:

- No one can predict the future.

- If I'm going to engage in "what ifs," I might as well choose healthy ones.

- If I believe in myself, I'll be able to handle any situation.

Filtering

If you are filtering out everything except the most negative aspects of a situation, you need to shift your focus. First, redirect your attention to active strategies you can use to make your situation more manageable. Look at the situation realistically rather than magnifying the negative aspects. Then, focus on the positive aspects of your situation. Examples of positive thoughts to counteract filtering out all but your negative thoughts follow:

- I can handle this situation.

- I've developed a number of resources to make this surgery turn out as positively as possible.

- I am undergoing this surgery for the positive reasons of . . .

- I'm looking forward to getting beyond the surgery and beginning to heal and recover.

- I've had the surgery and now I can focus on getting better.

Black-and-White Thinking

Thinking in black and white terms sets you up for disappointment because it doesn't allow for the possibility of *gradual* improvement. The first step in changing black-and-white thinking is to identify when you are using absolute words such as *all, every, always, never,* and *none*. The second step is to focus on how your situation may be changing in gradual steps. Last, remember that you always have a range of options, not just the extremes of black and white. The following examples will help you to avoid thinking in black-and-white extremes.

- I am making progress in the following areas

- My *ultimate* goal is . . . and I'm moving towards it in the following ways . . .

Overgeneralizing

When you overgeneralize you take one element of a situation and apply it to everything else. Stop overgeneralizing by reminding yourself to evaluate each aspect of a situation independently and realistically. Examples of counteracting overgeneralizing follow:

- I've been able to get through a lot of awful situations before, and I'll get through this one.

- Just because my last hospitalization was unpleasant, doesn't mean this one has to be as bad.

Mind Reading

Nobody can read another person's mind, although we all have a tendency to act as though we can. This may cause us to respond to others in ways that are based on inaccurate conclusions. For instance, you might think, "I know my doctor doesn't like me" based simply on your "mind reading" abilities. Remember, you *cannot* read another person's mind. Remember to check out the *reality* by reminding yourself of the following:

- I can't be sure about what he/she thinks unless I check it out.

- I need to act based on the facts, not on what I *assume* the facts to be.

Shoulds

If you find yourself using the words *should, ought, must,* you are discrediting either yourself or others by unrealistic standards. "Should" statements tend to lower your self-confidence and self-esteem. To know when this is happening, ask yourself the following questions: "Is this standard realistic?" "Is this standard flexible?" and "Does this standard make my life and situation better?" Then, remind yourself of the following statements:

- I do not have to be perfect.

- I will forget the shoulds, oughts, and musts and remember that I am doing the best I can.

- I am doing what I can to get better and I will reward myself for that.

Blaming

If you tend to blame yourself, remember that you tried to make the best choices at the time, whatever the outcome, and that you can continue to make healthy choices in the future. If you blame others, assess realistically how they went about making their choices, then remind yourself of those aspects of the situation that are in the realm of your control and responsibility. The following statements will help you to stop blaming yourself and/or others:

- Even though that guy caused my injury, I'm responsible for what happens from here on.

- I did the best I could.

- They are doing the best they can.

Summary of Healthy Self-Talk

The following examples illustrate the process of identifying negative self-talk and your responses to it and of substituting positive coping thoughts.

Stressful Situations

Contemplating any of the following situations could be very stressful and could cause you to engage in negative self-talk.

- The strange hospital surroundings

- The loss of independence

- Isolation from other people

- The surgery itself

- Pain—before, during, and after the surgery

Negative Self-Talk

The following examples are typical of the kinds of negative self-talk that prospective surgery patients find themselves doing, and the types of negative self-talk these thoughts are

- I can't stand the strange sounds, machines, and people in the hospital. The last time I was even near a hospital it was awful. (*overgeneralizing, catastrophizing*)

- I won't be able to do anything for myself in the hospital and after I come home. (*catastrophizing, filtering*)

- What if I don't have enough visitors, or too many? (*catastrophizing*)

- If the surgery doesn't take the pain away, it will be a failure and I will suffer for no reason at all. (*catastrophizing, black-and-white thinking*)

- I won't be able to stand the pain. I have a very low tolerance for pain and I should be able to handle it better, but I can't. (*shoulds, catastrophizing, self-blame*)

- I don't think my doctor likes me because he never smiles. (*mind reading*)

Emotional Response

The usual emotional response to such types of negative self-talk are as follows:

- Anxiety

- Fear

- Anger

- Depression or grief

Physical Response

The usual physical response to such negative self-talk is increased physical tension, which is manifested by the following symptoms:

- Shortness of breath

- Rapid, shallow breathing

- Increased heart rate

- Increased adrenalin flow

- Increased muscle tension

Positive Coping Thoughts

The following statements will help you to counteract negative self-talk and the emotional and physical responses that negative self-talk engenders.

- I can use distraction techniques to cope with the situation.

- I can ask for an explanation of the machines and procedures that will be used.

- I can gather information on how I can take control while I am in the hospital.

- I can determine before the surgery who will visit me and who will not.

- The surgery is being done to obtain the positive outcomes of . . .

- I can discuss with my doctor how pain control will be managed based on what I learn in this book.

Use the log below to develop your own list of positive-coping, self-talk messages.

Stop, Challenge, Reframe Self-Talk Journal

Use the following spaces for each entry. On the first line write down the situation; on the second line write your emotional response; on the third line write your physical response; and on the fourth line write your coping self-talk thoughts.

Situation: _____

Emotional response: _____

Physical response: _____

Coping self-talk: _____

Situation: _____

Emotional response: _____

Physical response: _____

Coping self-talk: _____

Situation: _____

Emotional response: _____

Physical response: _____

Coping self-talk: _____

Situation: _____

Emotional response: _____

Physical response: _____

Coping self-talk: _____

Situation: _____

Emotional response: _____

Physical response: _____

Coping self-talk: _____

Situation: _____

Emotional response: _____

Physical response: _____

Coping self-talk: _____

Affirmations

Affirmations are another method for helping you to cope with situations surrounding a surgery or another stressful medical procedure. Affirmations are similar to the coping thoughts we have previously discussed but they can be less related to the surgery experience itself. Affirmations are statements that "reaffirm" you and your abilities. They are positive statements about your self-worth, value, and dignity as a human being. People often confuse their self-worth and value with external circumstances such as financial success or physical appearance. Affirmations focus on real values.

The guidelines for writing affirmations are the same as those for writing coping thoughts. In summary, affirmations should be

- Short, simple and direct

- Written in the present tense

- Believable

Examples of some general affirmations follow. You can use these as a starting point for developing your personalized list of affirmations.

- I am responsible for and in control of my life.

- Life is an adventure.

- I am a valuable and unique person.

- I can handle it.

- I have a right to all of my feelings.

- It is OK to be myself.

- I can accept myself as I am.

- I am peaceful.

- I can learn to handle difficult situations.

- I look forward to new opportunities.

- I trust my capacity to overcome tough problems.

- I am learning to balance important aspects of my life.

Once you have developed your list of affirmations it is important to "work" with them on a regular basis. We recommend that you write the list of affirmations on an index card and keep it with you for periodic review. You can also tape it somewhere you will see it throughout the day. You should review your affirmations, possibly out loud, at least four or five times a day. It can be helpful to review them when you start your day and just before retiring at night. Take your list of affirmations with you to the hospital and use them when you are recovering.

PART IV

Mind-Body Techniques

Part IV focuses on developing your mind's influence over your body.

Chapter 7 describes *stress* and the body's response to it, particularly in the medical environment. More importantly, it also describes the *relaxation response* and how it subdues the effects of the *stress response*. The chapter then offers a complete regimen for achieving the relaxation response, first through the practice of deep breathing, and then by cue-controlled relaxation.

Chapter 8 offers further techniques for achieving deep relaxation through imagery or visualization. It also touches on the value of distraction, humor, and hypnosis in relaxation and pain control.

Chapter 9 explores the ways in which music produces physical responses, and how it is used therapeutically.

Chapter 10 considers the role that spirituality and faith have long played in emotional and physical well-being, and how they can influence the healing process.

7

Relaxation Techniques

Surgery is a stressful event for both the body and the mind. Anxiety and stress are normal responses to surgery and can have such negative effects on your surgical experience as heightened emotional distress (anxiety, depression, anger), increased pain, slower healing, and more intense side effects. The stress response causes physical reactions such as decreasing the activity of your body's immune system, which slows healing and decreases your ability to fight off infection. (See Chapter 1 for a discussion of the surgical stress response.)

The stress of surgery does not begin with the surgery, nor does it end there. It actually begins from the moment you decide to undergo a surgery (anticipatory anxiety) and extends in some form until you recover from the operation. This surgery preparation program teaches you effective techniques for managing this tension.

What Is Stress?

It is important to have a good understanding of what stress is and what it can do to your body and mind. This chapter provides a solid rationale for the benefits of relaxation training.

Stress is generally defined as a physical or mental "demand" that is made on the body. Certainly, having a surgery falls within this definition. The body's stress response may include:

- Increased blood pressure

- Increased heart rate

- Increased muscle tension

- Rapid breathing

Did You Know That Many Medical Problems Are Caused by Stress?

Scientific studies suggest that up to 85 percent of all medical problems are caused by stress. This is not to say that the physical problem is "in your head." Rather, prolonged stress causes physical changes in your body that result in various medical conditions such as headaches, back pain, sleep problems, digestive disorders, and high blood pressure. Stress can worsen virtually any medical problem (or medical procedure such as surgery).

When you are tense, your body produces stress hormones to give you an energy burst. If you are in danger, these hormones help your body perform at maximum efficiency for survival reasons (the "fight or flight response"). But, when these hormones are released inappropriately over a long time, they damage the body. Being "stressed out" a lot is analogous to running your car's engine at high speeds. It may enable your car for a quick get-away, but will blow up the engine if done continuously.

The release of stress hormones is detrimental before, during, and after your surgery. The relaxation response will stop this response and cause the release of biochemicals helpful to your healing and recovery.

- Release of stress hormones

- Reduced blood flow to the head, gut, skin, hands, and feet

These physical correlates of stress (also called the stress response) can hamper your response to surgery. Learning how to activate the relaxation response is the key to overcoming these stress symptoms. The stress response and the relaxation response are completely incompatible. If you learn to elicit the relaxation response, the stress response can be effectively blocked. Also, the relaxation response provides many benefits beyond simply blocking the stress response. It actually enhances your body's ability to heal.

The Relaxation Response: More Than Just Relaxing

It is important to distinguish between the relaxation response and simply relaxing. In discussing relaxation training as part of the preparation for surgery program, patients often ask if they can simply do something they enjoy such as listening to music or quietly sitting in the backyard. Although these activities are certainly relaxing, they do not necessarily elicit the relaxation response.

The type of relaxation that is important in preparing for surgery is the relaxation response, a specific physiological state which is the exact opposite of your body's condition when it is under stress. The relaxation response was first described by Dr. Herbert Benson and his colleagues at Harvard Medical School in the early 1970s. The relaxation response may produce these physical changes:

- Decrease in heart rate

- Decrease in respiration rate

- Decrease in blood pressure

- Decrease in skeletal muscle tension

- Decrease in metabolic rate and oxygen consumption

- Decrease in analytical thinking

- Increase in the brain's alpha wave activity

The relaxation response can only be achieved through regular practice of a relaxation technique. Once you have learned to elicit the relaxation response, you will notice that you feel more relaxed in other areas of your life, even when you are not directly practicing the relaxation technique. Table 7.1 provides a direct comparison of the physiological effects of the stress response versus the relaxation response.

Table 7.1
A Comparison of the Stress Response and the Relaxation Response*

Physiologic State	Stress Response	Relaxation Response
Metabolism	Increases	Decreases
Blood pressure	Increases	Decreases
Heart rate	Increases	Decreases
Rate of breathing	Increases	Decreases
Blood flowing to the muscles of the arms and legs	Increases	Stable
Muscle tension	Increases	Decreases
Alpha (slow) brain waves	Decrease	Increase

*Adapted from Dr. Herbert Benson, 1996.

Learning how to achieve a relaxation response produces many benefits associated with directly managing the stress of surgery and enhancing postoperative healing and recovery, as well as with other aspects of your life. These are summarized as follows:

- Reduction of generalized anxiety

- Prevention of the buildup of cumulative stress

- Increased energy level and productivity

- Improved concentration, memory, and ability to focus

- Reduction of insomnia and fatigue; deeper and more restorative sleep

- Prevention or reduction of such stress-induced physical disorders as high blood pressure, migraines, tension headaches, asthma, and ulcers

The Power of Ancient Meditation Techniques

Dr. Herbert Benson was one of the first scientists to study the meditation techniques of Tibetan monks. His expeditions and investigations resulted in the publication in 1975 of his book, *The Relaxation Response*. Since that time, he has continued to investigate the meditation techniques of various groups.

Dr. Benson and his colleagues at Harvard Medical School have made some amazing observations during the course of their studies. For example, his team documented that monks could actually dry icy, wet sheets on their naked bodies in temperatures of 40°F! Within three to five minutes of placing the dripping sheets on their skin, the sheets began to steam. Within thirty to forty minutes the sheets were completely dry.

In another observation, monks from monasteries in Ladakh were able to survive a night outside wearing only thin wool shawls and sandals. They were at an elevation of 19,000 feet and the temperatures were at or below zero.

In each of these findings, the monks were able to elicit the relaxation response to the highest level. This demonstrates the powerful potential these techniques have for augmenting our physical and mental capacities. Dr. Benson identified two simple steps for eliciting the relaxation response:

1. Repeat a word, sound, prayer, phrase, or muscular activity, and

2. Passively disregard everyday thoughts that come to mind, and return to the practice of your repetition.

• Increased awareness of your actual emotional state and feelings. (Being tense and "stressed out" dulls awareness of your actual feelings which can impede the surgical process.

The relaxation response also directly impacts on the physical stressors associated with surgery. These benefits include:

• Pain reduction

• Control of nausea

• Enhanced immune response that may promote faster healing

• Improved respiratory function that may reduce the possibility of pneumonia

There are many techniques and exercises for bringing about the relaxation response. These include breathing techniques, progressive muscle relaxation, visualizing a peaceful image, meditation, and others. In our experience, we have found breathing exercises to be the easiest way to learn to elicit the relaxation response and probably the most appropriate technique for preparing for surgery. The exercises are straightforward and require very little body movement. This makes them useful in almost any type of surgery, even those which place some restriction on movement or position during recovery. In fact, respiratory therapists often help patients breathe more effectively during their hospital recovery. Generally, the breathing techniques presented here create no problems and have been used successfully in our preparation for surgery program.

Different Types of Breathing

It may seem strange to discuss learning how to breathe properly because breathing is essential for life, and we often take it for granted that we are doing it properly. In reality, very few people actually breathe in the healthiest fashion. Breathing in brings oxygen into your lungs, where it enters your blood. When the blood leaves your lungs through the arteries, it has a high oxygen content. It is pumped by your heart to all parts of your body, delivering the essential oxygen to other cells and exchanging it for carbon dioxide. The blood is then pumped back through your heart and returned to the lungs where the carbon dioxide is expelled by breathing out. Once the carbon dioxide is released by the lungs, they take in fresh oxygen again, and the cycle repeats itself. Improper breathing can cause an insufficient amount of oxygen to reach the blood cells, and poorly oxygenated blood is one aspect of the stress response.

There are generally two types of breathing: *chest breathing* and *abdominal* or *diaphragmatic breathing*.

Chest Breathing

Chest breathing, also termed "shallow breathing," leads to poorly oxygenated blood, as discussed above. In chest breathing, with each in-breath (inhalation) you expand your chest, raise your shoulders, and tuck in your abdomen. The breaths tend to be shallow and brief. They also can be quite irregular and rapid.

Chest breathing can be associated with high anxiety states in which you may experience holding your breath, hyperventilation, shortness of breath, constricted breathing, or the feeling that you are going to pass out. You are more prone to chest breathe when you are under stress, which in turn decreases your ability to cope with the stress.

Extreme cases of chest breathing can produce a hyperventilation syndrome due to exhaling an excess of carbon dioxide in relation to the amount of oxygen you are taking in. The symptoms of hyperventilation include a rapid heartbeat, dizziness, tingling sensations at the fingertips and around the mouth, feeling nervous and jittery, and disorientation. Learning how to breathe abdominally will help to alleviate these symptoms.

Abdominal or Diaphragmatic Breathing

Abdominal or diaphragmatic breathing is the way we breathe naturally. Newborn infants are abdominal breathers, as evidenced by the movement of their stomachs with each breath. Also, adults breathe abdominally when they sleep. Unfortunately, most of us learn over the years to be chest breathers, so that learning to breathe diaphragmatically may seem unnatural at first. Diaphragmatic or abdominal breathing is, however, the most natural, healthy, and beneficial way to breathe.

The diaphragm is a sheetlike muscle that stretches across your chest and separates the chest cavity from the abdominal cavity. The diaphragm muscle usually expands and contracts automatically, although it can be controlled voluntarily. When inhaling, the diaphragm contracts downward, causing air to be pulled into the lungs and pushing the abdominal wall outward. When exhaling, the diaphragm and chest relax, the lungs contract, and the air is forced out. As this process continues, your abdomen once again flattens out and the cycle starts over. Breathing diaphragmatically or abdominally allows you both to take a deeper breath and to exhale more completely.

Learning how to breathe diaphragmatically is a key component of learning how to elicit the relaxation response.

How to Elicit the Relaxation Response

The remaining section of this chapter will guide you through an easy-to-learn technique for eliciting the relaxation response. To do this you will need to do three things:

1. Assess how you now breathe.

2. Practice breathing exercises regularly.

3. Make time to practice.

This section presents more information about breathing techniques. We have outlined several breathing/relaxation exercises to help you develop the relaxation response.

Breathing Exercises

By regularly practicing proper breathing techniques, you can learn to elicit the relaxation response. In this section, we review several types of breathing exercises adapted from the *Relaxation and Stress Reduction Workbook* (1995). But first, you must assess the way you breathe now.

Breathing Awareness

The following is a four-step exercise to help you become aware of how you normally breathe. Complete the following exercise:

1. Lie down on your back in a comfortable place. (If lying on your back is not comfortable, you may try sitting or reclining in a chair.)

2. Place one hand on your breastbone, which is underneath your collarbone, and the other hand over your belly button. Close your eyes.

3. Without trying to change your normal breathing, become aware of which part of your body moves as you inhale and exhale. The hand on your breastbone will monitor chest breathing and the hand over your belly button will monitor abdominal breathing. Take several breaths and pay attention to your body's movements. Now, which hand rises when you inhale? The one placed over your belly button or the one resting on your chest?

4. If your belly button moves up and down with each breath, you are breathing diaphragmatically. If your chest moves up and down with each breath, then you are more of a chest-breather.

In the space below, record what you observed from the above exercise. You will return to this section after practicing the breathing exercises. That will help you to monitor your progress in learning how to breathe abdominally.

_____

_____

_____

_____

Diaphragmatic or Abdominal Breathing

The following exercise will help you to develop the skill of abdominal breathing. Practice it until you are confident that you can breathe abdominally during a relaxation session of five to ten minutes.

1. Lie down in a comfortable position on your back with your legs straight and slightly apart. Allow your toes to point comfortably outward and let your arms rest at your sides without touching your body. Place your palms up and close your eyes.

2. Focus your attention on your breathing and place your hand on the spot that seems to rise and fall the most as you inhale and exhale. Notice the position of your hand. Is it on your chest, your abdomen, or somewhere in between?

3. Now, gently place both of your hands (or a book) on your abdomen and focus on your breathing again. Notice how your abdomen rises as you inhale and falls as you exhale. Try to make your hands rise and fall as you inhale and exhale.

4. Breathe through your nose during this exercise. (You may need to clear your nasal passages before you begin.)

5. If you have difficulty breathing into your abdomen, press your hand down on your abdomen as you exhale and allow your abdomen to push your hand back up as you inhale deeply. The pressure of your hand makes you more aware of the movement of your abdomen as you breathe.

6. Notice whether your chest moves in harmony with your abdomen, or seems rigid. If the latter, take a few minutes to focus on the movement of your abdomen and concentrate on allowing your chest to follow its natural motion.

7. If you have difficulty with the above exercise, you might try the following alternative. Lie on your stomach with your head resting on your hands. Take deep abdominal breaths so that you can feel your abdomen pushing against the floor as you breathe.

8. As you practice abdominal breathing for five or ten minutes, scan your body for muscle tension, tightness, or trembling.

Deep Breathing

After you have mastered abdominal breathing, this deep breathing exercise can help you to achieve the benefits of the relaxation response discussed at the beginning of this chapter.

It can be practiced in several positions, but the following one is recommended:

1. Lie down on your back. Bend your knees and move your feet about eight inches apart with your toes turned slightly outward. This will help straighten your spine and keep you comfortable as you practice the breathing exercise. If you have back problems, you may want to place a pillow under your knees for extra support. If you are unable to lie on your back, sit in a comfortable, supportive chair or recliner.

2. Mentally scan your body for any tension.

3. Place one hand on your abdomen and one hand on your chest.

4. Inhale slowly and deeply through your nose into your abdomen, so that your hand rises as much as feels comfortable. Your chest should move only a little and should follow the movement of your abdomen.

5. When you feel at ease with Step 4, practice the deep breathing cycle. While smiling slightly, inhale deeply and diaphragmatically through your nose. Then, exhale through your mouth by gently blowing the air out of your lungs and making a gentle "whooshing" sound like the wind. This will help to relax the muscles of your mouth, tongue, and jaw.

6. Take long, slow, deep breaths that raise and lower your abdomen. Focus on the sound and feeling of breathing as you become more and more relaxed.

7. Continue this deep breathing pattern for five or ten minutes at a time, twice a day. Once you have done this daily for a week, try to extend your deep breathing exercise periods to fifteen or twenty minutes.

8. At the end of each deep breathing session, scan your body again for tension. Compare the tension you feel at the end of the exercise with that you felt at the beginning of the exercise.

9. As you become more proficient at deep breathing, you can practice it at any time during the day, in addition to your regularly scheduled sessions. Concentrate on your abdomen moving up and down and the air moving in and out of your lungs.

10. Once you have learned to use deep breathing to elicit the relaxation response, you can practice it whenever you feel the need for it.

Breath Counting

A common tendency in first learning the breathing techniques presented in this chapter is to pace the breathing cycle (inhale—exhale) too fast. This exercise helps you to pace your breathing properly.

1. Sit or lie in a comfortable position, as in the previous exercises.

2. Breathe in deeply using the diaphragmatic technique you learned in the previous exercises. After you fill your lungs completely, pause before you exhale—then exhale *fully*. As you exhale, allow your entire body to just "let go."

3. To ensure that your breathing is slow and rhythmic, slowly count to four as you inhale (1, 2, 3, 4) then slowly count to four as you exhale. Pause briefly at the end of each inhalation.

4. Notice that as you count slowly, your breathing gradually becomes slower and your body relaxes more fully. As you continue to practice this exercise, your mind will also become more clear and relaxed.

Cue-Controlled Relaxation

Cue-controlled relaxation is a powerful technique that can be used either alone or in conjunction with deep breathing. In cued relaxation you learn to use a cue to signal the relaxation response. Although the cue can be anything, it is usually a muscular signal or a verbal signal, such as a word. To use a word or phrase, say something quietly to yourself, such as "relax." We recommend a muscular signal, such as gently touching your thumb and index finger together, rather than a verbal signal.

To use cue-controlled relaxation with this signal, you simply touch your thumb and forefinger together when you want to elicit the relaxation response. This is especially useful when you find yourself in a situation where you can't actually engage in deep breathing. For example, when you are talking to your doctors or having an uncomfortable procedure performed on you, it is possible to gain control over stress and pain by signaling yourself with a cue to relax.

How Does Cue-Controlled Relaxation Work?

In order to understand how a cue, such as speaking a word or touching your fingers together, can cause relaxation, we will briefly review one of the most important findings in twentieth-century psychology. In the early 1900s, Ivan Pavlov, a Russian physiologist, conducted a series of experiments that demonstrated how basic physiological responses can be controlled by totally unrelated cues.

In these famous experiments, Pavlov showed that the salivation response in dogs can be activated by the sound of a bell. Normally, the salivation response in mammals is caused by the sight and smell of food—that is, when food is present, the salivary glands produce saliva to aid in the chewing and digestive processes. Since bells have nothing to do with the salivation response, how can they cause salivation? Pavlov found that by repeatedly ringing a bell when the dogs were fed, the sound of the bell became associated with the presentation of food and would cause salivation even when no food was present.

This form of learning is called a *conditioned response* or *Pavlovian* or *classical conditioning* and occurs daily in many aspects of our lives. For example, like the bell, even a thought can be the cue to elicit a conditioned physiological response. If you simply think about biting into a lemon, you may experience some salivation. The thought, or visual image, of a biting into a lemon is associated with past experiences of tasting actual lemons and has thus become a cue to activate the salivation response. Another example of classical conditioning can be seen in patients who have become nauseated following the injection of a drug. After this experience they may find themselves becoming nauseated by the smell of the alcohol that was used to clean the skin prior to the injection. This can occur even though the alcohol smell originally had nothing to do with their nausea.

In cue-controlled relaxation, a cue is also employed to elicit the relaxation response through classical conditioning. The cue, such as the word "relax," a phrase, or touching your fingers together, is analogous to the bell in Pavlov's experiments. The cue is associated with the deep breathing that elicits or causes the physiological changes associated with the relaxation response. Eventually, with practice, the cue elicits the relaxation response in the same way that the bell caused salivation. Note that typically the cue will not result in the same degree of relaxation as actually doing the breathing, but in some situations you don't need to be deeply relaxed. You may only need to stop stress, anxiety, and pain from escalating, and in this case cue-controlled relaxation can be very effective.

How to Learn Cue-Controlled Relaxation

The following steps will help you to learn cue-controlled relaxation, if you first have a basic mastery of deep breathing and eliciting the relaxation response. Practice deep breathing for at least a week before beginning to work with cue-controlled relaxation. Follow these steps:

STEP 1: Choose a Cue

The cue you choose can be verbal or muscular. Verbal cues include words such as "relax," "breathe," or the number "one"; phrases, such as "I am Calm," or a phrase from a prayer. An easy muscular cue is to gently touch the thumb and index finger of your nondominant hand together. You can even combine several cues, though we favor the simplicity of using only one. Although many patients prefer to use a verbal cue, we encourage the use of the finger cue because it is easy to use, especially in situations where you are interacting with others or engaging in thought processes that make the use of verbal cues difficult.

STEP 2: Conditioning the Relaxation Response to the Cue

Whenever you practice the deep breathing exercise, use the last twenty breaths at the end of your practice session to learn cue-controlled relaxation. For example:

Word or Phrase Cue If you choose a word cue, such as "relax," stretch out the sound of the word while you are exhaling by saying "reeelaax." With practice, simply saying "relax" to yourself will result in relaxation.

Finger Cue If you choose the finger cue, gently squeeze your thumb and forefinger together on the inhalation, or in-breath, then relax the squeeze on the out-breath. You don't need to part the thumb and forefinger when you relax the squeeze. The action should be effortless—squeeze and release very gently. The cue, then, is simply to squeeze your thumb and forefinger together, not too tightly, and then release the squeeze when you want to signal the relaxation response. The finger cue is discrete, can be used anywhere, and does not interfere with social interactions or thought processes. Again, this is our method of choice and we recommend that you try it.

Uses of Cue-Controlled Relaxation

Cue-controlled relaxation can be used in many situations where it is difficult or impossible to engage in deep breathing, or when you need to slow down and redirect your attention to relaxation. Examples of uses for cue-controlled relaxation follow:

To signal the relaxation response in any situation. Cue-controlled relaxation can be used in any situation, especially if it is difficult to do deep breathing. For example, if you are in a stressful meeting with your doctor discussing medical matters and you want to reduce your distress, deep breathing would be conspicuous and disruptive, but cue-controlled relaxation would be helpful.

To refocus your concentration on breathing, relaxing, and coping. If you are in a situation where you cannot relax and are beginning to feel distress, the cue can be used as a signal to relax and focus on taking care of yourself.

Thought stopping. Cue-controlled relaxation is a powerful technique for stopping or disrupting negative and unproductive thoughts. For example, imagine that you are getting carried away with negative thoughts which are causing you to feel anxiety or distress. The cue can be used to disrupt or stop these thoughts and redirect your thinking toward coping self-statements.

To prepare yourself for an uncomfortable medical procedure. Cue-controlled relaxation is an excellent way to prepare yourself for an uncomfortable medical procedure, especially when doing deep breathing is difficult or impossible. Employing a cue either to prepare for or to cope with a painful medical procedure is one of the most effective uses of cue-controlled relaxation. For example, you can use the cue to signal relaxation to reduce the discomfort associated with such procedures as a nerve block, an injection, or the placement of an IV catheter. The cue is especially effective if the procedure interferes with deep breathing, as in the removal of a nasal gastric tube passing through the nose into the stomach.

To manage acute pain. Cue-controlled relaxation can be used to manage episodes of sharp pain following your surgery. Recovery from some surgeries may be characterized by episodes of acute (sudden onset) sharp pain. The cue can be used to get you through these episodes if you use it as soon as you experience the pain.

To control nausea and vomiting. Nausea and vomiting are among the most distressing effects of surgery and anesthesia. Use cue-controlled relaxation the moment you feel the first sensations of nausea to reduce its impact, as well as to disrupt the negative thoughts that often accompany nausea and vomiting and that increase distress.

In summary, cue-controlled relaxation is a very powerful skill that can be used in a variety of situations related to your surgery and in everyday life. As with all of the skills presented in this book, you must take time to practice! The cue will work for you, but only if you practice using it to elicit the relaxation response.

Guidelines for Practicing relaxation

As in learning any new skill, the relaxation exercises must be practiced to be effective. The following guidelines will help you establish a regular practice regimen. They will also help you to get the most out of each breathing session. The learning process will require more time initially, but as your skills improve, less practice time will be needed.

1. **Twice a day.** It is important to practice the breathing exercises twice a day to learn how to elicit the relaxation response.

2. **Quiet location.** Practice your breathing exercises in a quiet location where you will not be disturbed or distracted. For instance, keep the phone from ringing and isolate yourself from distracting noises outside. You can use a fan, air conditioner, or recordings of nature sounds to mask outside noise.

3. **Give a five-minute warning.** It can be useful to give yourself and other family members a five-minute warning before beginning your breathing exercises. This can help you take care of "loose ends" that might cause interruptions. If you are worried about a number of things you have to do, it may be helpful to make a short list to free your mind from the distraction of trying to remember what you need to do after your exercise is finished.

4. **Practice at regular times.** It is important to set up regular practice times, as this will make you more likely to follow through on your deep relaxation exercises. Choose times that don't conflict with other demands on your time. Don't practice when you are so tired that you are likely to fall asleep (for instance, right after a big meal or just before bed).

5. **Practice on an empty stomach.** After a big meal you may be more likely to fall asleep while trying to relax. Also, the process of digestion after a meal can disrupt the relaxation response. Therefore, we recommend that you practice on an empty stomach, if possible.

6. **Assume a comfortable position.** Assume a comfortable position for practicing your relaxation exercises. A common position is lying flat on your back with your legs extended and your arms comfortably at your sides, but some medical conditions may not allow this posture. You can also practice the breathing exercises while sitting or standing, or while supporting your body in ways that increase your comfort. For instance, if you have back problems you may find that the most comfortable position is lying flat on your back with your knees supported by a pillow. If you are tired or sleepy, you may need to practice the exercises sitting up rather than lying down so that you don't fall asleep. It is important to become *deeply* relaxed *without* falling asleep.

7. **Loosen your clothing.** It is helpful to loosen any tight clothing and take off your watch, shoes, glasses, jewelry, and any other constrictive apparel. Again, the object is to be as comfortable as possible while you practice the exercises. Also, these exercises often rely on breathing in through your nose, so clear you nasal passages before practicing the exercises.

8. **Set your worries aside prior to practicing.** Set aside your worries before you begin your relaxation exercise. Using the five-minute warning technique can be helpful in this regard. During the five-minute warning write down all of the things that are on your mind. This will allow you to better focus on the relaxation exercise, as those other concerns will be documented for your attention once you finish the exercise.

9. **Assume a passive attitude.** As you begin the relaxation exercise, adopt an attitude of "allowing" the relaxation response to happen. Don't try to relax or control your body and don't judge your performance. Just focus on your breathing, and relaxation will occur on its own.

Obstacles to Practicing

Almost everyone who practices the relaxation exercises finds the relaxed state quite enjoyable and beneficial. Certainly, experience has demonstrated that the ability to elicit the relaxation response can be very useful in preparing for surgery, during the hospitalization time, and during recovery. Even so, almost everyone comes up against common obstacles to practicing the relaxation exercises on a regular basis. As stated previously, regular practice is essential to learn how to elicit the relaxation response so that when you need it you can use it.

Some of the most common obstacles (or excuses) to practicing relaxation on a regular basis are discussed below.

There Is No Time to Relax

"I don't have time to relax." This is probably the most common obstacle to practicing the relaxation procedures. What this statement really means is that you have not placed a high priority on practicing the relaxation exercises. Ask yourself why you have not found the time to practice on a regular basis. It may be that you have given other activities higher priorities than taking care of yourself. You *must* choose to practice on a regular basis, knowing that the outcome will be an improved response to your entire surgical experience.

It's Boring

Some people have trouble with the relaxation exercises because they find them "boring." Often, these are people who must be constantly busy and feel particularly anxious when they try to relax or close their eyes. If you have experienced this situation, ask yourself why you have trouble just "being still" with yourself. Although some of these issues are discussed in other chapters, the more common reasons include negative self-talk such as the following:

- I only feel worthwhile when I am doing something. (*black-and-white thinking*)

- I feel others will think I am being irresponsible if I take time out for myself. (*mind reading*)

- I must keep busy all of the time. (*shoulds*)

- I know it is important to take the time to do these exercises, but I have too many other responsibilities. (*filtering/Yes-butting*)

I Don't Have a Place to Relax

When people have trouble practicing the relaxation exercises on a regular basis, one common excuse is that they don't have a place to relax. They often find that the house is too noisy or that there are other demands on their attention, such as job responsibilities, the needs of others, child care, etc. Even in these situations, you can structure your environment to give yourself twenty minutes a day to practice the exercises. To make your home easier to practice in, try some of the following procedures:

- Put the phone on an answering machine and unplug the phone in your bedroom.

- Give your family a five-minute warning that you will be unavailable for the next twenty minutes while you practice the exercises.

- During the five-minute warning period, be sure that family demands are placed on hold or managed by another household member.

- Close the door to the room in which you are going to practice, and place a "Do Not Disturb" sign on the door knob.

- If there is not room enough to get away from household distractions, you may have to practice when the other people in the household are out of the house.

In the following space record any obstacles you may be confronted with and a solution to each.

_____

_____

_____

_____

_____

_____

_____

Peculiar Sensations When Practicing Relaxation

A small number of people, especially those not accustomed to relaxation due to feeling "speeded up" most of the time, may experience either peculiar sensations or anxiety when they practice relaxation. If this is true for you, start out slowly and keep your practice sessions short initially. As you practice more, gradually work up to longer periods of practice until you reach the target of about fifteen or twenty minutes. Generally we do not recommend practice for more than thirty minutes at one time.

Mind Chatter

At times it may be difficult to keep your mind focused on the breathing exercises. Your mind may wander to other issues of the day or become distracted by outside noises or negative thoughts. This is common and is nothing to worry about. The following can be helpful for managing mind chatter:

- Allow yourself to "notice" the distracting thought or issue and let it "pass through" your awareness knowing that you will have plenty of time to deal with it later

- Use the more active breathing techniques such as breath counting to keep your mind focused

- Use the imagery exercises discussed in Chapter 8

- Write down all of your worries or "to dos" during the five-minute warning.

- Set a timer to go off if you find yourself worrying about how much time has passed during the practice periods

What Is Meditation?

Meditation differs in scope and practice from the relaxation and imagery approaches described in this book. Meditation is a discipline with twenty-five-hundred-year-old roots in Buddhism and Hinduism. It takes many different forms, as do the spiritual practices of Judaism and Christianity.

Increasing numbers of medical programs incorporate meditation techniques into their treatment of medical- and stress-related problems. Dr. Jon Kabat-Zinn, a professor of medicine at the University of Massachusetts Medical Center (UMMC) and founder of its pioneering Stress Reduction Clinic, has used meditation with thousands of patients suffering from hypertension, heart disease, AIDS, chronic pain, cancer, diabetes, and stress-related disorders, to mention a few. This innovative program includes sessions in mindful- ness meditation, which differs from more familiar forms of meditation, such as Transcendental Meditation (TM), that involve focusing on a mantra, phrase, or prayer to minimize distracting thoughts.

In mindfulness meditation, instead of ignoring distracting thoughts or sensations, including physical discomfort, you focus on them. Unlike all Western medicine approaches, the focus is not on symptom reduction. Rather the aim is for patients to cultivate greater awareness and wisdom, and to learn to live each moment of their lives as fully as possible, no matter how painful it may be. The results of this program have been very impressive and well documented in several scientific publications (Kabat-Zinn 1990 and 1993).

(Continued on following page)

Another well-known program incorporating mind-body techniques in the treatment of medical and stress related problems is offered by the Mind/Body Institute, in Boston, Massachusetts. Its founder, Dr. Herbert Benson, Associate Professor of Medicine at Harvard Medical School, is a pioneer in the use of meditation techniques for treating many different medical and stress related conditions. His book, *The Relaxation Response* (1975), is recommended.

There are additional meditation references in the resources section.

Precautions

Using breathing exercises to elicit the relaxation response is both safe and natural, but there are some instances that require precautions related to the body's need to adjust to being relaxed. These include such problems as seizure disorders, insulin-dependent diabetes, and hypertension.

In seizure disorders, some seizures are brought on by a change in the arousal level, such as going to sleep or waking up. Because the brain waves that take place during relaxation are similar to the brain waves of some sleep stages, people with sleep-onset seizure disorders may experience seizures when they first start practicing the exercises. Discuss this issue with your doctor. Our experience indicates that the triggering of these seizures generally subsides with continued practice or through the choice of alternative relaxation techniques.

In rare cases, patients who are on insulin may find that their insulin requirement decreases through regular practice of the relaxation exercises. Again, discuss the serious issue of hypoglycemic reactions with your doctor.

Certain medications such as antihypertensives and antidepressants may interfere with normal blood-pressure adjustments when changing posture or position. For instance, you may feel light-headed or dizzy when you rapidly stand after lying down. Therefore, change your posture slowly after practicing the relaxation exercises. For instance, you should slowly go from a lying down to a sitting position, giving your body time to adjust. Then, slowly move to a standing position. This prevents any drop in blood pressure that might be caused by rapid postural changes.

Use the following Relaxation Log to track your exercises until they become a regular part of your routine. Simply record each time you practice the relaxation response as well as any comments or problems related to the practice session. You can also record the cue you have selected to associate with relaxation. Note that Chapters 8, 9, and 10 contain techniques you may wish to include in your relaxation practice sessions.

Relaxation Log

Record the day and date of each session. Practice at least twice a day, ten to twenty minutes for each session. Also, record positive aspects of each session (e.g., very peaceful, enjoyable images, used a prayer), as well as any problems that arose (e.g., interruptions, falling asleep, intruding thoughts).

Day and Date   *Comments/Problems*

_____

_____

_____

_____

_____

_____

_____

_____

_____

_____

_____

_____

_____

8

Imagery and Visualization

Imagery and visualization are powerful techniques that are essential components of a preparation for surgery program. In this chapter, we first present techniques for learning the effective use of imagery and visualization. We also discuss how distraction and humor help cope with surgery.

Imagery and visualization are terms that are used interchangeably. In this discussion, we simply refer to both of these techniques as imagery. Imagery is nothing magical. In fact, you engage in imagery every day. It is thought to be one of the basic ways in which your mind stores information in the unconscious. When you daydream or dream while asleep, these unconscious images are accessed. Imagery is used in athletic training—you might imagine "in your mind's eye" the golf ball landing on the green before you hit the shot or the basketball going through the hoop before you make the free throw.

Using imagery techniques to promote physical healing dates back hundreds of years. From a very early time, it has been known that the thoughts and images that arise from our imagination can have very real physiological consequences. In fact, sometimes our brains cannot differentiate between an experience of something that is really occurring and an imagined image.

There are many examples of this in day-to-day life. Think about the last time you watched a scary movie. During the course of the movie, you may have noticed your heartbeat and respiration increasing, your breathing accelerating, and your palms becoming sweaty. All of these were very real physical responses to events that were *not* real. The movie simply activated your *imagination*, to which your *body* responded.

Another example of your body responding to your imagination is found in dreaming. When you experience a nightmare you react physically as if it were actually happening. Also, a dream about a very pleasant experience may evoke strong physical and emotional reactions, and an erotic dream can evoke a sexual physical response.

These observations demonstrate that imagination is, in fact, a normal thought process. The power of the imagination has been demonstrated in many areas of health care. Specifically, imagination can have such positive effects as:

- **Achieving fuller, deeper relaxation.** This is the use of imagery as a relaxation technique. Imagery most often employed after the initial relaxation state is achieved through the practice of the breathing exercises described in Chapter 7.

- **Enhancing physical healing.** Many imagery exercises are designed to activate the body's natural ability to heal itself. Such images might include white blood cells attacking and dissolving germs, or injured tissues receiving valuable nutrients from increased blood flow.

- **Relieving pain.** Imagery can help you to remove yourself from the experience of pain while it is occurring. Using imagery techniques, you can mentally put yourself in another place to decrease the perception of pain and discomfort. Also, there are more specific images for reducing the experience of pain such as turning the volume down on your pain or changing the imagined red color of your "ball of pain" to a more relaxing color, such as blue.

- **Improving sleep.** Sleep disturbances are common when you are anticipating surgery, in unfamiliar hospital surroundings, or recovering at home after surgery. Imagery to promote restful sleep may often involve a "passive" technique in which you imagine your body feeling the physical sensation of relaxing (e.g., "warm and heavy").

- **Promoting muscle relaxation and decreasing anxiety.** The images may be of your muscles "unwinding" like the knots in a twisted rope, a "ball of tension" in your body dissipating each time you exhale, or your muscles becoming smoother and looser.

- **Providing distraction from a stressful medical procedure.** This type of imagery is very effective when you are undergoing the discomfort or pain of an unpleasant medical procedure. Guided imagery, in which you "guide" your imagination through a sequence of events such as walking on the beach or down a forest path, is a particularly powerful way to distract your mind.

As you can see from these examples, imagery can be used in many health situations, including the surgery process. This chapter will specifically focus on imagery for surgery and healing.

Guidelines for Practicing Imagery

The Following are guidelines for developing an effective imagery exercise. Read all of the guidelines and imagery examples in order to decide which imagery approach might work best for you. Then develop your own powerful imagery exercises. Remember that imagery is a natural process and that you are always in complete control, as if you are a movie director and can project whatever image you want onto your mental screen.

Tape-Record Your Imagery Exercise

Recording your imagery exercise on audiotape can promote your regular relaxation practice and make your imagery experience as powerful as possible. (Using a tape recording is also useful for developing the relaxation response elicited by the breathing exercises discussed in Chapter 7.)

First write out your imagery script including places where you will pause. Be sure to include the breathing techniques from the previous chapter as part of your script. Then record the script onto a tape for use in regular practice. When making an audiotape of this type, it is important to read through the script very slowly and pause at times. Speak in a calm, comforting, and steady pace, letting your voice flow in a smooth and somewhat monotonous manner, but without whispering. The examples of imagery exercises described later in this chapter will help you get a feel for where to pause when taping your script.

Use Familiar Images

Our clinical experience and some research studies suggest that it is most effective for you to develop an image with which you are quite familiar. Generally, you will find it easier to conjure up all aspects of the image if you have actually experienced it in the past. For instance, you should choose a beach or forest scene where you have enjoyed a pleasurable visit. Images developed from your own memory don't have to derive from a single remembered experience but can be drawn from bits and pieces of different memories. In the following section some standard imagery exercises are presented that can be modified to fit your own personal experiences.

What Is Distraction?

Distraction is defined as turning one's attention away from an original focus to another focus. Clinical experience and research have shown that distraction can be a powerful technique for managing stressful medical procedures and for controlling pain. Distraction techniques for these purposes involve focusing your mind on something other than the stressful event. This decreases the impact and intensity of the stressor. The imagery exercises in this chapter provide one method of distraction by keeping your mind busy and turning your attention away from pain.

You may discover your own distraction techniques for coping with medical stressors. For example, some patients who have undergone uncomfortable stressful medical procedures, employed such distraction methods as counting the holes in ceiling tiles, repeating words or poems, singing and humming, engaging in conversation, and whistling.

Other distraction techniques may include staring at a stationary object or spot on a wall (focal point), tapping the rhythm to a song with your finger or foot, and listening to music.

Use All Five Senses to Develop Your Image

Your image is most powerful if you develop it using all five of your senses—sight, sound, touch, smell, and taste. For instance, if you are imagining a beach scene to relax, observe the view of the ocean and beach, remember the smell of the seaweed, the sounds of

Humor and Your Health

A cheerful heart is good medicine.
Proverbs 17:22

Laughter and humor are not only fun but can improve your mood, reduce emotional tension, exercise your cardiovascular system, and promote social interactions. Beyond these obvious benefits, research has shown that there may be a physiologic basis for the conclusion that laughter is good medicine. Drs. David Sobel and Robert Ornstein (1996) have summarized studies that have demonstrated that laughter can provide such health benefits as decreasing sensitivity to pain, improving sleep, and boosting the immune system.

They suggested that you can use humor for health in the following ways:

- Expose yourself to humor through films, joke books, and comic radio and television shows.

- Keep a humor journal in which you record funny thoughts or experiences.

- Tell jokes to others and be able to laugh at yourself.

- Look for the funny side of stressful situation. Sometimes laughing about a stressful situation is the only control you can exert, so you might as well try to have fun with it.

- Spend time around happy, optimistic people.

As can be seen, humor can help you cope with the process of going through a surgery.

seagulls and the waves crashing, the salty taste of the ocean air, and the feel of walking on the warm sand with your bare feet.

Use a Pleasing Image

The old adage that one person's feast is another person's poison applies to imagery as well. Using imagery is a very personal and individualized experience, and should be pleasing to you.

As an example of the importance of individualized images, consider the standard relaxation image called "The Beach Scene." Although many people find this relaxing, others may find it distressing. We were reminded of this while leading a group relaxation/imagery exercise. We chose the beach scene as a standard image for the group to develop. At the end of the exercise, we asked the group members to comment on their experience with the image. Although most found it pleasant and very relaxing, one woman felt it was distressing and anxiety-producing. She said that she absolutely "hated" going to the beach. For her, a trip to the beach meant not being able to find a place to park, suffering through a sunburn, eating sandwiches gritty with sand, and listening to a radio with bad reception. There was no part of the beach scene that she found relaxing.

This example illustrates that you must develop your own image to create an imaginary scene that will work for you.

Sneak Up on the Image

Attempting to focus on an entire complex set of images at one time may be difficult and stressful. This creates a problem especially when you are trying to use the imagery to manage a stressful situation. Margo McCaffrey, R.N. (1989) has suggested that it can be helpful to "sneak up on the image."

To avoid becoming frustrated in creating the scene, sneak up on the image by constructing it slowly. For example, if you have chosen a forest scene as your image, begin by imagining that you are at home preparing to go to the forest, or that you are driving to the forest. Imagine arriving at the trail head, getting out of the car, and slowly walking into the beautiful mountain scene which is the goal of your final image. Sneaking up on the image helps you to relax and adopt an attitude of "letting it happen," rather than trying too hard.

Use One Image at a Time

Try to visualize only one total image at a time. Trying to maintain several images at once is stressful and usually does not accomplish the goal of imagery, which is to relax.

Precede the Imagery with a Relaxation Exercise

Use a relaxation exercise, as described in Chapter 7, *before* you begin to visualize your chosen image. Although not required, this can greatly facilitate the imagery exercise. Choose one of the breathing exercises and practice it until you are skilled at eliciting the relaxation response. Then add an imagery exercise as described in this chapter. Each session of relaxation and imagery should last about ten to twenty minutes. All of the guidelines discussed in Chapter 7 for practicing the relaxation exercises also apply to visualizing an image in order to relax and distract your mind away from stressful thoughts or events.

Practice the Image

It is important to practice imagery regularly to develop this skill, just as in developing any other skill such as riding a bike or playing an instrument. The ability to create a mental image using all five senses may be difficult at first but it does improve with practice. If your images are not initially vivid, don't worry about it. As you practice, you will notice more details coming into focus, along with the growing feeling that you are actually in the image. As discussed above, a tape recording of your image can facilitate practice sessions.

Ending Your Image

Develop a technique to bring your image to a close without stopping it abruptly. A common side effect of using imagery is a slight sense of drowsiness afterwards. You can avoid this by using a technique for ending the image. One common method is to count silently from one to five, then, on the last count, to inhale deeply, open your eyes, and say to yourself, "I feel alert and relaxed."

Here is another example of an ending statement:

In a moment, I will notice myself becoming more alert, refreshed, and awake. As I count from one to five, I will become more awake, renewed, and energized. When I get to five, I can open my eyes, feeling refreshed. One . . . gradually becoming more alert . . . Two . . . becoming more and more awake . . . Three . . . beginning to slowly move my fingers, hands, and arms . . .

How Do You Handle
Medical Phobias?

There are certain aspects of the medical environment that are known to be particularly anxiety-producing for a significant number of people. One example of this is the common fear of needles and injections. Another example is undergoing an MRI scan. In this painless procedure you must lie very still in a large tube while the machine takes its "pictures." The machine makes a banging sound while it is operating. Approximately 10 to 20 percent of people find this so stressful that they cannot complete the test.

Systematic desensitization is a technique for helping people to overcome phobias or "irrational fears." It allows you to get accustomed slowly to what you fear. First, you learn how to elicit the relaxation response and use the methods for countering negative thoughts. Second, you make a list of situations related to the fear from the least frightening to the most fearful. For example, you might imagine getting ready to go for an MRI, arriving at the MRI center, going into the exam room, lying on the table, hearing the thumping sounds, and finally going into the tube. Third, you practice imagining each item on the list during your relaxation exercise. You imagine the first item on the list while staying relaxed. Then, when you are able to imagine the first item without experiencing distress, you move to the second item, and so on. It is important to stay relaxed as you move to the next item.

(Continued on following page)

Four . . . almost back to an alert state . . . I can now begin to move my toes, feet, and legs . . . and . . . Five . . . opening my eyes and finding myself fully awake, alert, renewed, and refreshed.

After completing an imagery exercise, get up slowly. Some people find that stretching after an imagery exercise is helpful, too.

Don't Worry If Your Image is Not Vivid

You can get the beneficial effects of imagery even if your image does not have great detail or is not particularly vivid. With practice the details of your images will emerge and you will begin to have a sense of actually being there. Do not judge your performance or make this exercise stressful in any way.

Incorporate Affirmations or Prayer into Your Imagery

As part of your imagery exercise, you can incorporate any of the affirmations or prayers discussed in Chapter 10. For instance, affirmations such as "I am letting go," "I am at peace," and "All of the tension is flowing from my body" are commonly used for relaxation and imagery training. Chapter 10 has some more helpful affirmations and also some focus prayers that are very helpful when used during imagery exercises.

Standard Imagery Exercises

The following imagery exercises are standard examples that have been developed over a number of years. These examples illustrate the use of the guidelines for developing imagery discussed above. You can use these examples if you like, or develop individualized and personal exercises. It is most beneficial to customize your image to your individual experience. In the examples, the dots represent pauses to give the exercise a slow pace.

At the end of this chapter there is a space for writing your own imagery script.

The References and Resources section contains resources for more specific information regarding this technique for handling phobias. See Bourne (1995) and Davis, Eshelman, and McKay (1995).

You can then tape record this script while speaking slowly. Once you have developed your relaxation and imagery tape, practice with it on a regular basis.

The standard imagery exercises presented here are called "Passive Muscle Relaxation," "The Beach Scene," "Pain Reduction," and "Ball of Healing Energy." For more information on these techniques, please refer to the Resources and References section. (See Achterberg (1985), Bourne (1995), Lusk (1992), and McCaffery and Beebe (1989)). For all of the following exercises, it is assumed that you will already have learned to use breathing to elicit the relaxation response. If you make a tape, record the breathing exercises at the beginning and then incorporate the imagery sequence after completing the breathing exercises. It is also important to end the image as previously discussed. In the first example script, all of these phases (breathing exercise, imagery, ending the imagery) are included.

Example Script: Passive Muscle Relaxation

When you are ready, allow your eyes to slowly close.... Take in a full, deep breath through your nose, allowing your lungs to fill completely. Let the air go all the way in, breathing down into the bottom of your lungs. Notice the cool sensation in your nose as the air rushes in.... Then, breathe out through your mouth while slightly pursing your lips.... Notice that the air you exhale is warm and moist.... Release all of the air in your lungs as you exhale completely.... Slowly repeat this cycle several times.... Breathing in through your nose and out through your mouth.... Remember, there is nothing else to think about except becoming completely and deeply relaxed....

(Pause three to five minutes here for the breathing exercise)

You may notice that the healthy breathing exercise has already helped you become quite relaxed.... As you allow yourself to relax more and more fully, begin to focus your attention on your fingers and hands.... As you mentally focus your attention on your fingers and hands, notice the sensations that are coming from them.... Notice your hands resting on another part of your body or elsewhere.... Simply focus on the sensations coming from your fingers and hands.... Imagine what it would feel like for your hands and fingers to become more and more relaxed.... Let go of any excess tension you may feel in your fingers or hands.

As you continue to relax and breathe peacefully, slowly move the focus of your attention to the sensations in your forearms and upper arms.... As your fingers and hands continue to relax, allow that feeling of relaxation to move into your forearms and upper arms.... You might notice your hands or arms feeling warm or heavy as they relax.... Or you may notice them feeling cool and light. . . . Simply focus on what the relaxation response feels like for you.

As your arms continue to relax with every breath, allow the feeling of relaxation to move into your head, neck, and shoulders. . . . Imagine what it would be like for your forehead to relax completely. . . . Allow the muscles around your eyes to relax. . . . As you relax the muscles of your jaw, you may notice that your lips separate slightly. . . . Allow your shoulders to relax completely. . . . Focus your attention on these parts of your body, and imagine letting go of any tension that you notice. . . . Just allow the wave of relaxation to extend throughout your arms and upper body.

When you are ready, focus your attention on the sensations coming from your stomach and back. . . . Again, notice how the relaxation response moves slowly down your body as you let go of any tension in your stomach and back. . . . Imagine what it would be like for all of the muscles in your stomach and back to loosen completely. . . . It is as if you are inhaling relaxation and exhaling tension with every breath. . . . There is nothing else for you to focus on right now except enjoying the feelings of relaxation throughout your upper body.

As you continue to enjoy those feelings of relaxation, imagine the pleasurable sensation moving into your upper legs. . . . Allow the relaxation response to move further and further down your body. . . . There's nothing else to focus on—just enjoy the relaxation response. When you are ready, allow the relaxation response to move further down into your ankles, feet, and all the way to your toes. Notice how relaxation spreads throughout all the muscles of your legs and feet. Again, you may notice your entire body becoming heavier and heavier, or lighter and lighter. You may also notice a tingling sensation as part of the relaxation response. . . . These are all normal sensations that are a part of relaxing. . . . Simply focus on what relaxation sensations feel like. . . . You may feel warmth or, perhaps, coolness. Enjoy the sensation of your entire body being deeply relaxed. As you relax further, take a few moments to enjoy the sensations of relaxation. . . .

(Pause here for one or two minutes.)

In a moment, you will notice becoming more alert, refreshed, and awake. Even so, remember you can call upon the relaxation response at any time you like throughout the day. . . . Simply take a deep breath and tell yourself to "relax" as you exhale. . . . This will recall the relaxation sensation. . . .

As I count from one to five, you will become more awake, renewed, and energized. When I get to five, you can open your eyes, feeling refreshed. One. . . . gradually becoming more alert. . . . Two. . . . becoming more and more awake. . . . Three. . . . beginning to slowly move your fingers, hands, and arms. . . . Four. . . . almost back to an alert state. . . . you can now begin to move your toes, feet, and legs. . . . and. . . . Five. . . . opening your eyes and finding yourself fully awake, alert, renewed, and refreshed.

Example Script: The Beach Scene

It is about five in the afternoon on a midsummer day. . . . You are walking along a shady path that opens up to a very beautiful and expansive beach. . . . As you walk from the path onto the sandy beach, you notice that it is virtually deserted. . . . The beach extends off in both directions farther than you can see. . . . The sun has not yet begun to set, but it is getting low on the horizon. . . . The sun is a deep and golden yellow, the sky is a brilliant blue, and the sand glistens white in the sunlight. . . . As you walk on the sand in your bare feet, notice it rubbing between your toes. . . . The sand is warm and comfortable. . . . Notice the taste and smell of the salt in the ocean air . . . . There is a residue of salt deposited on your lips from the ocean spray. . . . You can slightly taste its presence. . . . Listen to the roaring sound of the surf as it rhythmically washes in and out from the shore. . . . Listen to the far-off cry of a seagull as you continue to walk along the beach. . . . Notice yourself becoming more and more relaxed as you continue walking down the beach. . . . You have nothing else to think about except enjoying this moment. . . . Feel the warm sea breeze blowing against your face, and the warmth of the sun on your body. . . . You feel more and more content as you enjoy the sights and sounds and scents of this beautiful beach. . . . As you walk, you see a sand dune that would be so comfortable to sit down and relax against. . . . As you sit, look out over the beach, the waves, and the sun on the horizon. . . . The sun has started to set, causing the sky to turn scarlet, pink, gold, orange, amber, and crimson. Allow yourself to settle firmly against the comfortable sand dune as you enjoy the sinking sun's reflection on the water. The sand forms perfectly to your body as you settle against the dune. . . . As you sit allow yourself to relax more and more. You find yourself relaxed, peaceful, and content.

Example Script: Breathing Out Pain

Continue to breathe comfortably and slowly, feeling your body relax more and more each time you breathe out. . . . If you wish, the next time you breathe in imagine that your breath goes directly to that part of your body in which you are experiencing pain or discomfort. . . . Imagine that your inhaling brings with it the valuable oxygen your body needs. . . . Your deep breath also brings with it a sense of calm and comfort. . . . As you slowly exhale, imagine that just a bit of the pain and discomfort is exhaled along with the air you breathe out. . . . As you exhale some of this pain and discomfort, the tissues left behind seem to be more relaxed, healthy, and comfortable. . . . At first, this reduction in pain may be only slightly noticeable, but it seems to become more noticeable with each breath. . . . Each time you breath in, imagine the air flowing to the area of pain and discomfort. . . . The air brings a sensation of health and comfort. . . . Then, each time you breathe out the air, notice the area of pain and discomfort becoming smaller and smaller. . . . As you breathe out, you are exhaling discomfort and pain. . . . Breathe in relaxation and breathe out pain.

Example Script: Healing Energy

As you continue to relax, focus once again on your breathing. Notice how you are slowly breathing in. . . . Feel the air going into your lungs. . . . Notice your lungs filling completely with air as you inhale. . . . Then, as you exhale notice the air rushing out of your lungs and mouth. . . . Enjoy the experience as you become more and more relaxed each time you inhale and exhale. . . . As you continue to relax, begin to imagine a ball of white light forming in the area of your chest and lungs. . . . This is a ball of healing energy. . . . It may not be particularly clear or distinct and that is perfectly fine. . . . Whatever its shape and texture, simply notice what your ball of healing energy looks like. . . . Focus for a few seconds on this ball of healing energy in your chest area. . . . When you feel ready, you may begin to notice this ball of white healing energy move to an area of your body that is feeling pain or discomfort. . . . Notice the ball of healing energy moving slowly to that part of your body. . . . Imagine that ball of healing energy settling in that part of your body As it settles there. . . . imagine it helping the tissues to become more and more healthy. . . . Imagine the white ball of healing energy bringing with it valuable nutrients and healing power. . . . As the power of the healing ball of energy begins to work, you might notice a warming or cooling sensation in that part of your body. . . . You might also notice a slight tingling sensation. . . . Simply focus on what the healing experience feels like as the ball of energy begins to work. . . . As you exhale, notice the ball of energy moving away from your body, taking with it toxins, tension, and injured tissue. . . . Each time you inhale, imagine the ball of healing energy moving directly to your area of discomfort with its healing energy. . . . Each time you exhale, notice the ball of energy moving away, taking with it some of the pain, discomfort, and tissue damage. . . . When you breathe in, it brings with it valuable relaxation and healing power. . . . Each time you breathe out, it removes discomfort, pain, and toxins.

Summary of Guidelines for Effective Imagery

The following statements summarize how to use the power of imagery effectively:

- Tape record your imagery exercise.

- Use a familiar image.

- Use all your senses to develop the image—sight, hearing, smell, touch, and taste.

- Use an image that pleases you.

- Sneak up on the image.

- Use one image at a time.

- Precede the imagery exercise with a relaxation exercise.

- Practice visualizing the image.

- Use a technique to end the image.

- Don't worry if the image is not vivid or detailed.

- Incorporate affirmations or prayer into the image.

Creating Your Own Imagery Exercise

In the following space, write down your own relaxation and imagery exercise:

_____

_____

Hypnosis

Hypnosis is a natural state of heightened, attentive, focused concentration and suggestibility that can make it easier to relax and to control your mind and body. We are often asked about using hypnosis in our surgical preparation program. Although we use hypnosis frequently when working with individual patients, we have chosen not to include it as part of this program for the following reasons:

- Hypnosis is best performed by a licensed health care professional (psychologist, physician, or dentist) with experience in surgical preparation. The focus of this book is on *self-management*, that is, doing the program yourself, and to have someone assist you with hypnosis is not consistent with this orientation. In addition, many of you may not have access to professionals who do hypnosis for surgery.

- There are widespread misconceptions about hypnosis that may interfere with its effectiveness. We review these misconceptions in this chapter.

It should be kept in mind that the surgical preparation program presented in this book is fully effective without the use of hypnosis. Basically, hypnosis is just another tool, similar to relaxation and imagery. We include this information here for those who wish to explore the use of hypnosis, and who do have access to appropriate professional assistance.

Hypnosis in Surgery

Hypnosis is a powerful technique that has had a cyclical history of acceptance and rejection since the time of Mesmer, over two hundred years ago. Today, it is widely used to treat many psychological and medical conditions. Hypnosis has proven especially effective in surgical preparation. It has been used to reduce surgical stress, to promote healing, and to control surgical pain (Hilgard and Hilgard 1983). Hypnotic suggestions have also been used to control intraoperative and postoperative bleeding, to promote postoperative digestion and bowel functioning, and to boost immune function (Bennett and Disbrow 1993). In fact, before the advent of anesthesia, hypnosis, along with alcohol, was the most effective means of controlling surgical pain.

Hypnosis is still used in circumstances where anesthesia cannot be used for reasons of safety or religious conviction. For example, hypnosis is used for minor surgical procedures such as a simple biopsy or incision. It is also used for major surgical procedures such as abdominal exploration, pneumonectomies, Caesarean sections, hysterectomies, thyroidectomies, prostatectomies, hemorrhoidectomies, skin grafts, and mammoplasties (Spanos, Nicholas, and Chaves 1989). It can be very useful during surgeries where the patient is under regional anesthesia and may be awake and aware of the surroundings. Hypnosis may also be used with patients undergoing uncomfortable and painful diagnostic procedures such as nerve blocks, catheter placements, laparoscopic examinations, colonoscopies, and MRIs. In dentistry, hypnosis is a well-established technique for controlling dental fears, pain, and bleeding. It is especially effective in the control of nausea and vomiting associated with surgery, medications, and chemotherapy.

One caveat to the use of hypnosis in medical practice is that more scientifically rigorous studies are needed to prove the many impressive claims made for it. There is controversy about whether you actually enter into a unique state of consciousness when hypnotized because researchers have been unable to clearly identify any unique patterns of physiological activity or brain waves to distinguish hypnosis from waking or relaxed states (Spanos and Chaves 1989). Whatever is happening, however, it is clear that researchers and clinicians consistently report benefits from using hypnosis.

Can I Be Hypnotized?

The experience of hypnosis is somewhat familiar to all of us. Doctors Orne and Dinges (1989) have listed a variety of naturally occurring hypnotic-like experiences that may give you an idea of what hypnosis feels like. Here are a few examples:

- You are in a room full of people, socializing and mingling with the group but feeling mentally far away.

- You can sometimes block out sounds so that they no longer intrude on your thoughts, or so that you don't hear them at all.

- You are in conversation with someone speaking directly to you, and you're nodding in agreement, but you're so lost in thought that you don't understand what they're saying.

- You are doing some routine task when your thoughts wander far away, and then, a few minutes later, you discover that you've completed the task without even being aware of working at it.

Some people are more susceptible to hypnosis than others. Measuring hypnotic susceptibility has been a topic of considerable scientific research for decades, and many hypnotic susceptibility scales have been developed. The Eye Roll Test is part of an eight—part Hypnotic Induction Profile (HIP) developed by Drs. David Spiegel and Herbert Spiegel (1978). The Eye Roll Test may help you determine whether or not you are susceptible to hypnosis. Please note that the reliability of this test is questionable when not administered by a skilled professional and when done in the present context. But give it a try anyway. You will need the help of a friend. First, take in a deep breath and roll your eyes upward into your head as far as you can. Next, begin slowly exhaling and closing your eyes while trying to keep your eyes rolled upward as high as you can, showing as much of the white your eyes as possible. Have someone watch yur eyes. The more white of your eyes and the less iris showing as you close your eyelids, the higher your hypnotice susceptibility is prsumed to be. Figure 1 shows how to score the Eye-Roll test. Scores range from 0 to 4, with 0 indicating low hypnotic susceptibility and 4 indicating high susceptibility. Individuals with scores ranging from 2 to 4 are good candidates for hypnosis.

In a study by Drs. Reeves, Redd, Storm, and Minagawa (1983), patients with far-advanced cancer underwent an experimental treatment in which the tumor was destroyed by radio frequency–produced heat. This caused severe deep pain which was unresponsive to dangerously high doses of narcotics, and even to anesthesia. Patients were classified as having

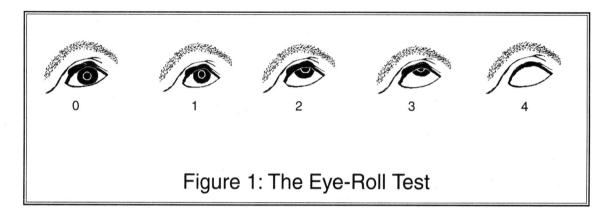

Figure 1: The Eye-Roll Test

high or low hypnotic susceptibility on *The Stanford Hypnotic Clinical Scale.* Half of the patients received two brief sessions of hypnosis with suggestions for pain control while the other half received no hypnosis. Only those patients who received the two sessions of hypnosis *and* were classified as highly susceptible to hypnosis achieved significant pain relief. Patients who received hypnosis but were classified as having a low susceptibility to hypnosis achieved little pain relief and fared no better than those who received no hypnosis. This study suggests that those who tend to be susceptible to hypnosis, as classified on standardized tests of hypnotic suggestibility, may benefit more from hypnosis than those who are not classified as hypnotically suggestible.

However, not obtaining a high score on a test of hypnotic susceptibility doesn't mean that you can't benefit from hypnosis. In the study by Dr. Reeves and his colleagues, patients were given only two brief sessions of hypnosis. It has been our experience that with more training, even those who are not classified as highly susceptible may benefit from hypnosis. Some clinicians believe that anyone may be hypnotized under the right conditions, and that failures reflect either poor hypnotic technique, resistance, or poor motivation on the patient's part.

The Hypnotic Procedure

The hypnotic procedure involves the following steps:

- *Relaxation*: Relaxation is first induced. Relaxed breathing, similar to that described in Chapter 7, is frequently used to do this.

- *Imagery*: Relaxing and healing images, similar to those described previously in this chapter, are presented to deepen the level of hypnosis.

- *Suggestions*: Specific therapeutic suggestions are then presented to address the needs of the patient, such as pain control.

Examples of suggestions for surgical recovery:

- You will be able to tolerate pain effectively and will need less medication. You will experience comfort and relaxation.

- Breathing comfortably and deeply makes you stronger. Your body is getting stronger and stronger.

- You feel a numbness moving into the painful area.

- Your wound will heal quickly. Blood will flow into the area and help you heal quickly.

- Your bowels and bladder will function promptly after surgery. Your stomach and intestines will begin to move and churn. You will be hungry and want to eat.

- You will feel calm and relaxed. You will have nothing to worry about. You can set your troubles aside until you heal.

- You will sleep soundly before and after the surgery.

- Your immune system helps heal your wounds and protects you against infection. It will be strong before and after surgery to help protect you. Your antibodies and white blood cells will carry away harmful bacteria. Your tissues will heal quickly. Your recovery will be speedy and complete.

Like the affirmations described previously in this chapter, you can make these suggestions as part of your surgical preparation program by repeating them when practicing the relaxed breathing and imagery exercises. If you choose to give yourself hypnotic-like suggestions, be sure and make them realistic. This process is known as self-hypnosis (Hadley and Staudacher 1989).

You may enter into light, medium, or heavy (deep) levels of hypnosis. A light level is associated with feelings of muscle relaxation and paresthesia (a tingling sensation on the skin), and hand levitation may be induced. At a medium level, pain is diminished and either partial or complete amnesia can be induced. A deep level of hypnosis is associated with auditory and visual experiences and deep anesthesia. Posthypnotic suggestions (suggestions presented during hypnosis to perform simple acts or feel certain experiences, such as pain control or enhanced healing, at a later time) are associated with deep hypnosis. Time can be distorted at all levels of hypnosis, but especially in deep hypnosis.

Misconceptions About Hypnosis

Widespread misconceptions about hypnosis, perpetuated by sensational stories in the media and movies, and unrelated to clinical use, have limited the use of hypnosis in clinical settings. Seven of the more common misconceptions are discussed by Drs. Pratt, Wood, and Alman (1984). These are

- *Hypnosis is a state of deep sleep or unconsciousness*: A person is not asleep when hypnotized. In fact, hypnosis is a state of relaxed attention where one is able to hear, speak, move around, and think independently. The brain waves of a hypnotized person are similar to those of someone who is awake. Reflexes, such as the knee jerk, which are absent in the sleeping person, are present when hypnotized.

- *Only gullible, weak-willed, or passive people can be hypnotized*: The reverse is true. Those who are most responsive to hypnosis tend to be more intelligent, creative, and strong-willed, because their powers of concentration are better. The main factor in benefiting from hypnosis is a strong motivation to participate.

- *Hypnosis allows someone else to control your mind*: This is perhaps the biggest misconception that dissuades people from pursuing and benefiting from hypnosis. Certainly books, movies, and stage hypnotists have capitalized on perpetuating this myth. People cannot be hypnotized against their will. Once hypnotized, a person cannot be forced or coerced into doing something they find objectionable or do not want to do. Suggestions presented to the hypnotized person are only as effective as the patient allows them to be. In fact, in clinical hypnosis people gain more, not less, control over their lives.

- *A hypnotized person might not be able to come out of a trance*: It is actually more difficult to become hypnotized than it is to slip out of hypnosis. Patients frequently become alert when a hypnotherapist stops talking, inadvertently says something inconsistent with the person's beliefs, leaves the room, or is otherwise distracted. If left alone when hypnotized, most people reorient, alert themselves, and awaken naturally.

- *A hypnotized person will give away secrets*: When hypnotized, a person is aware of everything that happens both during and after hypnosis, unless he or she wants to accept and follow specific suggestions for amnesia. Thus, secrets cannot be forced from a person unwilling to divulge them.

- *I probably cannot be hypnotized*: Some people are more responsive than others to hypnosis, but nearly everyone can achieve some level of hypnosis and can benefit from it with practice. Stumbling blocks to hypnosis include trying too hard, fears or misconceptions about hypnosis, and unconscious desires to hang on to troublesome symptoms. A licensed psychologist, physician, or dentist experienced in hypnosis can help a person overcome these stumbling blocks.

- *Hypnosis is a quick, easy cure-all*: This misconception is the opposite of the notion that hypnosis is mysterious, controlling, and dangerous. However, it is equally detrimental because extravagant and inaccurate claims result in a loss of credibility for hypnosis. While many have achieved remarkable results from hypnosis, others have not. When the focus is on a person's long-term problems, the course of hypnotherapy can be long and complex.

We want to emphasize that there are *no reported cases of harm* resulting from hypnosis. If you are interested in using hypnosis as part of your preparation for surgery program we recommend that you seek professional help from a *licensed* health care professional (psychologist, physician, or dentist) who has special training in medical hypnosis and experience in surgical preparation. You can obtain more information about hypnosis from The American Society of Clinical Hypnosis, and The Society for Clinical and Experimental Hypnosis, listed in the References and Resources section.

9

Music for Surgery

Music has the power to influence our thoughts, emotions, and physical state (Maranto 1993). For instance, the music of a marching band energizes most people; the national anthem makes you feel proud and connected; and a lullaby may induce calm and quiet. Beyond these common responses, music can also evoke individual, personal responses. There may be a special song or melody that evokes very specific thoughts, emotions, and images every time you hear it.

Music and Healing

The use of music in medicine (music therapy) has been developed over the past fifty years. Music therapy has been used in such diverse medical areas as neurological disorders, coronary care, cancer therapy, psychology, rehabilitation, and surgery. Music has been used to help patients throughout the entire surgery experience; before, during, and after their operations.

Here, we will consider some general findings regarding music and health, and then present guidelines for using music in your own preparation for surgery program.

The Familiarity of Music

Music is an emotional experience to which we all respond, but certain kinds of music will cause specific, personal emotional reactions. You may have a very positive and uplifting reaction to a song that someone else finds disagreeable. Moreover, the same music can induce different emotional reactions at different times. A melody may make you feel joyful at one time and sad at another time, and it may be difficult to predict which emotional reaction you will experience.

The Positive Effects of Music in Surgery

Dr. Cheryl Dileo Maranto (1993) has summarized research studies that suggest the positive effects of music on surgical outcome:

- Patients receiving music during surgery show better psychological, behavioral, and physiological outcomes than those not receiving music.
- Music may reduce preoperative anxiety in patients of all age groups.
- Postoperative music may decrease pulse rate and stabilize blood pressure.
- Listening to music reduces stress hormone levels during surgery.
- Music reduces the amount of general anesthesia needed for surgery.
- Music affords patients under regional anesthesia less need for postoperative analgesics and sedatives.
- Music and positive suggestion improve sleep and reduce pain, anxiety, and the level of analgesic use in patients undergoing heart surgery.

In considering its therapeutic value, you might be inclined simply to choose music that you regularly enjoy, such as country western, classical, rock and roll, jazz, gospel, etc. Although this might make sense intuitively, experience has shown otherwise. In fact, music that you often enjoy listening to may be the worst choice of music to aid you in your experience with surgery.

The Structure of Music

The structure of music affects our emotional and physiologic states. Most often, melodies have a beginning, a middle, and an end. If you know the melody, then you know how it will progress and how it will end. When listening to familiar music you unconsciously anticipate each part of the melody and wait for it to develop. This process of anticipation and waiting creates tension in the mind and body until the melody ends. This same phenomenon also can occur even if you don't know a particular melody and are hearing it for the first time. Composers know how to create tension in the listener as the structure of the music builds and resolves.

This anticipation, waiting, and tension are pleasurable emotional experiences under the right circumstances. However, when trying to become completely relaxed as when trying to elicit the relaxation response, this type of tension is counterproductive. For surgical patients, the musical structure of most melodies creates tension, not relaxation.

The Sounds of Music

Obviously, music is made up of sounds. The characteristics of the sounds of music, just as its structure and familiarity, affect our emotional response. Important elements of sound include tone, pitch, and loudness (decibel level). All of these should be considered when choosing music for surgery.

Loudness, or intensity, of sound is measured in decibels. When measuring loudness, 1 decibel is the lowest level of sound the normal ear can detect. For comparison, the loudness of a dripping faucet is about 40 decibels, that of an average alarm clock is 80, and that of a jet engine on take-off is 140. When you consider that these values follow a logarithmic scale, in which an increase of 30 decibels represents a thousandfold increase in acoustical power, you can see that our sense of hearing must adjust to an enormous range of loudness, in music as well as in all the other sounds that surround us.

Tone (timbre) and pitch are other characteristics of sounds that affect our emotional reactions. We are all familiar with the "fingernails on a chalkboard" phenomenon. This is a high-pitched sound that can make your hair stand on end. A certain tone or pitch at sufficient loudness can actually cause pain.

The Rhythm of the Music

The rhythm of the music is its beat. The beat can be fast or slow, regular or irregular. Music with a fast beat is energizing while music with a slow beat is calming. There is some indication that our natural heart rate of about 72 beats per minute is the dividing line that determines whether music is energizing or calming. Music with a tempo above 72 beats per minute may activate us while music with a tempo below 72 beats per minute may calm us. The consistency of the beat also affects our emotional and physical response to the music. Specifically, an irregular and inconsistent rhythm or beat can be quite disturbing and make us uneasy.

Can Patients Hear During Surgery?

Dr. Henry Bennett (1993) and others have suggested that patients may perceive sounds and conversations subconsciously during surgery. There is also some evidence that the nature of these conversations can have a postsurgical impact on the patient. For instance, a comment by a surgeon such as "These are the worst arteries I've ever seen" may be perceived by the patient and negatively affect recovery.

Dr. Henry Bennett suggests that the message to surgeons is simple—be aware of comments made during the surgery about the patient's condition. He also suggests that patients can avoid hearing negative messages during surgery by wearing earplugs or listening to relaxing music from a tape or CD player with headphones. Listening to a tape of positive relaxing and healing suggestions during surgery may even help the postoperative recovery.

It should be noted that, as compelling as the idea is that patients can hear during surgery, other scientists have been unable to demonstrate this (Eich, Reeves, and Katz 1985). Regardless of this controversy, there can be no harm in using techniques to prevent hearing during surgery.

Habituation to Sound

"Habituation" is a fancy word that simply means getting used to or becoming accustomed to something. Our senses have an amazing ability to habituate to the point that we do not notice stimuli that we are experiencing regularly. For instance, we will no longer notice a rancid smell after being exposed to it for a period of time. Similarly, we become accustomed to irritating and tension-producing sounds after being exposed to them for some time. Over time and repeated exposure, our brains actually block out the sensory input. In your home there may be noises that bothered you when you first moved in but that you no longer notice (e.g., highway noise, the hum of the refrigerator, or dripping water). The same may be true of noises that you experience at work.

The hospital environment is full of disturbing and tension-producing sounds such as people working around you and talking, patients coughing and calling out requests, machines humming, bells ringing, paging systems squawking, and the bustling of the operating room. For the people working in the hospital these sounds may not necessarily produce tension because they are completely habituated to them. But for you the experience could create considerable tension. Music therapy can help you manage the sounds of the hospital setting.

Anxiety-Reducing (Anxiolytic) Music

Stress-reducing or anxiolytic music is music, or musical sounds, arranged in a way that reduces anxiety and tension by taking into account the familiarity, musical structure, and tonal characteristics of the sounds.

Anxiolytic music is designed to be unfamiliar to the listener, so that it will not evoke negative emotions, thoughts, or memories. It avoids songs, lyrics, and singing, and the entire spectrum of familiar music from Gregorian chants to classical to rock.

Anxiolytic music also avoids melody, which, as discussed previously, can create tension through anticipation. Music without melody is a blend of sounds that allow the listener to relax completely.

Anxiolytic music uses some special characteristics of sound to achieve its therapeutic effectiveness. For example, the decibel level of the music is kept low, and tension-producing qualities of pitch and tone are avoided, as are abrupt changes in sound that could cause uneasiness.

Furthermore, anxiolytic music has either a slow, consistent rhythm or no rhythm at all. The slow-flowing, continuous motion of this sound fosters mental and physical relaxation because it does not create anticipation, waiting time, or tension. It does not begin, build, and end but rather seems to be endless.

Practical Guidelines

Based on the factors reviewed above, the following guidelines are suggested for choosing music to reduce anxiety and stress:

1. Use music that is unfamiliar to you in order to avoid negative associations.

2. Use music that does not have a melody.

3. Use music with relaxing properties of loudness, tone, and pitch.

4. Use music with a calming and consistent rhythm or beat, or with no rhythm at all.

You can obtain specially produced audiotapes of anxiolytic music. Some of these are designed specifically for coping with the surgery process. The most comprehensive packages include music to be used before surgery to deal with anticipatory anxiety, during surgery to block out the sounds of the operating room, and after surgery to enhance healing and recovery. The series of tapes by Linda Rodgers is listed in the References and Resources section.

10 ◯

Spirituality, Faith, and Healing

According to a Gallup poll conducted in 1990, 95 percent of all Americans said they believe in God, and 76 percent said they pray regularly. The pollster, George Gallup Jr., reported in an interview that, "Nine out of ten adults pray to God; nearly all who pray believe their prayers are heard and answered." (1990) These statistics underscore the fact that the vast majority of Americans recognize and accept the existence of a Supreme Being and are involved in a spiritual relationship with that Being through prayer. We would therefore be seriously negligent if we did not address the issues of spirituality, faith, and healing in a book about preparing for and recovering from surgery. For many people, a deep spiritual commitment and/or faith are the central focus of their lives and the key elements in managing various stressors.

If you already have a spiritual or religious commitment, the material in this chapter may be redundant to your experience. Even so, it may help you to reinforce your spiritual practices, especially in the face of such a major stressor as surgery. Those who do not have such a focus, and who believe that spirituality and faith are not relevant to surgery, may choose not to incorporate the material in this chapter into a preparation and recovery program. Throughout this book the program is individualized to include those elements that work for you as a unique person.

This chapter is based on the work and ideas of many authors. More information about any of these issues can be found in the books and articles listed in the References and Resources section. With that introduction in mind, let's explore how spirituality, religion, faith, and prayer can be important elements in your preparation for and recovery from surgery.

Religion and Spirituality

Religion can be defined either as:

1. Belief in a divine or superhuman power or powers to be obeyed and worshiped as the Creator and Ruler of the universe, or

2. Expression of this belief in conduct and structured ritual.

To be religious is usually characterized by adhering and conforming to a structured religion (e.g., Judaism, Hinduism, Buddhism, Protestantism, Catholicism, Islam, etc.). Spirituality is often thought of as something distinct from religion. Spirituality is a much broader concept. Though difficult to define, spirituality pertains to a deeply held belief in the individual's connection with others. It may include an awareness of and relationship with a higher power or supernatural being apart from the structure of the belief or worship. Thus, a person may be spiritual without necessarily being religious. Or, someone can exhibit religiosity (religious behavior) without necessarily being very spiritual. In this chapter, we use the term "spirituality" to refer to both religious and spiritual behaviors.

There are many terms for the "Higher Power." These include God, the Almighty, the Supreme Being, the Infinite Absolute, the Alpha and Omega, Jehovah, the Maker, the Holy One, the Blessed One, the Divine, among thousands of others. In this chapter, we refer to God, or higher power. Regardless of the term we use, it is doomed to inadequacy as a descriptor. When trying to represent God within the finite limits of language, humans have always been frustrated. St. Anselm, who lived between 1033 and 1109 A.D., expressed the problem as "God is that, the greater-than-which cannot be conceived."

Spiritual Commitment and Health

In spite of the nearly universal belief in God and in the efficacy of prayer, in the realm of medical treatment and the delivery of health care, including surgery, these aspects of the patient's life are rarely taken into account.

The Doctor-Patient Spirituality Gap

A recent magazine article discusses that, despite the desires of patients, their doctors are reluctant to talk to them about faith as a factor in their medical care and healing. The following table, adapted from *Time* magazine (Wallis 1996), shows the results of a telephone survey of 1,004 adult Americans. These results provide more evidence of the importance to patients of faith and prayer in the area of medical issues and health.

	YES	NO
Do you believe in the healing power of prayer?	82%	13%
Do you believe praying for someone else can help cure their illness?	73%	21%
Do you believe God sometimes intervenes to cure people who have a serious illness?	77%	18%
Do you believe in the ability of faith healers to make people well through their faith or personal touch?	28%	63%
Do you believe doctors should join their patients in prayer if the patients request it?	64%	27%

Consistent with these findings, Dr. Larson, a professor of psychiatry and behavioral sciences at Duke University Medical School, says that, in the medical profession, there is a lack of significant understanding of the importance of religion and prayer to many patients. He states that, "We aren't talking about proselytizing or force-feeding patients religion, but responding to positive effects such as the hope, coping, and peace they feel prayer brings" (Larson 1993). Even though you may have made a significant religious or spiritual commitment in your life, it is unlikely to be addressed or acknowledged by your doctor or surgeon.

On the other hand, Dr. L. Dossey (1993) has argued that patients may not want to bring their spiritual beliefs into their relationship with their doctor. So, bringing the spiritual part of your life into your doctor-patient relationship will probably depend on you, but it may also depend on whether your doctor is comfortable with discussing these matters. If your spiritual beliefs are important to you, you can help your doctor understand their value to you in the management of your surgery. Here are some suggestions to help in this regard:

1. If you are religious, tell your doctor. Most doctors will not ask.

2. Help your doctor understand that your beliefs are important to you and relate to your surgery. Do not, however, expect your doctor to focus on your spiritual needs, although this may vary depending on your doctor's own beliefs.

3. Have realistic expectations about your doctor's role. He or she will focus first and foremost on your medical treatment or surgery, and may acknowledge your spiritual values simply by being a good listener. If spiritual issues arise, it will probably be incumbent upon you to update your doctor.

4. Consider consulting a religious or spiritual counselor with whom you feel comfortable. His or her advice and counsel can supplement your medical care.

Assert Your Spiritual Needs

Don't feel too timid or embarassed to ask your doctors about any special spiritual needs that you feel need to be met. The following illustrates this point:

Nina, a forty-six-year-old woman, was scheduled for a complete hysterectomy in one month and had many fears about the impending operation. Although she was raised in the Jewish tradition, she drew much personal strength from her spiritual practice of Hindu meditation. She considered herself a "Hin-Jew." She wanted to be able to rely on her spiritual practice during the stress of surgery and recovery. She wanted to listen to a taped recording of her special mantras while in the hospital and to have a very small altar in her room. She was hesitant to ask for these because her doctor was Christian, and she would be operating on her in a Jewish hospital where there was a mezuzah placed at the entrance to every room. Nina wasn't sure that her Hindu meditation would "play well" in that environment. However, she also realized that she needed to continue her spiritual practice during the surgical period. So, she mustered enough courage to ask her surgeon and a hospital representative if they could meet her requests and honor her spiritual needs. Much to her surprise they agreed!

She recorded her mantras on a small portable cassette tape player and used a pair of lightweight earphones for listening. Upon arriving at the hospital the morning of her surgery, she listened to the mantras continuously, and the anesthesiologist continued to play the tape throughout her surgery and in the recovery room. (NOTE: If you choose to listen to a tape for a long period of time you will need an auto-reverse player. Also attach an extra set of batteries and any special instructions to the cassette player with tape.)

In addition to the taped mantras, her brother was able to set up a small table in her room as an altar, where she placed a picture of her guru and some flowers. Nina's surgery and postoperative course of healing went exceptionally well. She attributes this to the strength she drew from being able to continue her spiritual practice during the entire surgical process.

Medical Science and Religion

The same lack of understanding of the importance of spirituality to many patients holds true for the scientific and medical study of religion and prayer. Some medical investigators believe that scientists are contemptuous of religious belief and rarely have made religious faith the focus of scientific study. A number of interesting studies substantiate this conclusion. For example, a review of over 1,000 articles in primary care physician journals revealed that only 1.1 percent of them (11 studies) assessed religious considerations (Orr and Isaac 1992). In another review, it was found that, of the hundreds of thousands of English medical journal articles published in the past 200 years, only about 200 studies investigated the role of faith (Levin and Schiller 1987). Dr. H. Benson (1996) concludes that these findings show "just how taboo God has become in the recent history of Western medicine."

In spite of the fact that, historically, both medical and scientific researchers have largely ignored the possibility that spiritual faith can have a positive effect on health, most people believe that this is indeed the case. More recently, scientific investigations have begun to document that there is a correlation between spiritual practices and healing and recovery.

Spiritual Beliefs and Health

Today scienctific and medical researchers are beginning to study mind/body/soul interactions. New research is being launched to investigate the effects of faith on health and healing. Evidence is mounting that there are significant health benefits to faith, spirituality, and prayer. The following summaries are just a few recent findings:

1. Dr. Jeffrey Levin reviewed hundreds of epidemiologic studies and concluded that belief in God lowers death rates and increases health (1994).

2. In a 1995 study, Dr. Thomas E. Oxman at the Dartmouth Medical School found that of 232 patients who had undergone elective open-heart surgery for either coronary artery

or aortic valve disease, the "very" religious were three times more likely to recover than those who were not.

3. In a study of hospitalized male patients, one in five reported that religion is "the most important thing that keeps me going." Also, nearly half of these patients rated religion as very helpful in coping with their illness. Religious coping behaviors helped these men to experience significantly less depression (Larson 1993).

4. In a seven-year study of seniors, religious involvement was associated with less physical disability and less depression (Larson 1993).

5. It has been found in various research studies that church attenders have lower blood pressure and nearly one-half the risk of heart attack as the general population, even after the effects of smoking and socioeconomic status have been taken into account (Larson 1993; Matthews 1994).

6. Of 300 studies on spirituality in scientific journals, the National Institute for Health Care Research found nearly three-fourths of these studies demonstrated that religion had a positive effect on health (Larson 1993).

7. In a study performed by Dr. Peter Pressman of Northwestern University Medical Center, thirty elderly women who were recovering from surgical corrections for a broken hip were interviewed to determine the relationship between their religious beliefs and health. Postoperatively, those who held strong religious beliefs were able to walk significantly further and were less likely to be depressed than those who had no religious beliefs (1990).

These findings validate what those who are spiritual have known all along: *Belief in a higher power makes a positive contribution to our physical health.*

The Benefits of Spiritual Beliefs

As can be seen from the above findings, religious and spiritual beliefs form a vital part of the way a majority of people view life and cope with problems. The following paragraphs summarize the benefits that these beliefs can provide:

- **A sense of meaning and purpose:** We all feel, to a greater or lesser degree, that it is important that our life has a purpose, a sense of meaning, or a sense of completeness. Spiritual beliefs can provide us with that sense of meaning and purpose and help us to rise above the distractions, problems, and sorrows of everyday life.

- **Setting healthy priorities:** Spirituality provides a framework in which to set priorities and place everyday stressors within a larger perspective. A spiritual connection can help us to maintain a sense of inner security and safety. When we feel that we are not alone in the universe, we can feel secure even when we are temporarily separated from our loved ones. A strong sense of inner security also results from the belief that there is no problem beyond the scope of God.

- **Comfort in the face of illness and crises:** Spiritual beliefs can provide great comfort in the face of major health crises, such as undergoing major surgery. The belief that a higher power can give us guidance and peace of mind is comforting in and of itself.

- **Security and safety:** A sense of security and safety is especially important when approaching a major life stressor such as surgery. Through a spiritual connection, the need for inner security can be met by the belief that a higher power is watching over you.

- **Peace of mind:** Peace of mind results from feeling secure and safe. When you place your trust in a higher power, you feel less fear, and you worry less about your ability to deal with life's challenges. Of course, approaching, experiencing, and recovering from major surgery is such a challenge. Peace of mind can be developed by "letting go" and "turning over" to a higher power the anxieties and fears associated with surgery. The phrase "Let go and let God do it" expresses this belief succinctly.

- **Self-confidence:** Self-confidence is developed and nurtured when you remember that you were created by a higher power and that you are a part of the universe of creation. Your belief in a higher power can also help you accept that you are worthy of love and respect, by virtue of the fact that you have been created.

- **Guidance:** Your relationship with your higher power can also provide you with guidance. Because your higher power is "all knowing," you can draw upon this wisdom when asking for guidance.

These are just a few of the benefits that a spiritual belief can provide when you are preparing for, going through, and recovering from a surgery. They are all related but you may experience some of these benefits more than others. Focus on those gifts that spirituality can give you. Remember, it is easy to lose spiritual focus when you are under stress—but that is the time when it is most important.

Prayer

Feeling connected to a higher power can be achieved in a variety of ways, including associating with people with spiritual beliefs, practicing religious rituals, and engaging in prayer. In this section, we focus on some general guidelines for prayer as they may relate to the spiritual component of a preparation for surgery program.

What Is Prayer?

It is beyond the scope of this book to discuss the various ways in which one can pray. The definition of prayer suggests two common forms: petition (asking something for one's self) and intercession (asking something for others). Other types of prayer include confession (the repentance of wrongdoing and asking of forgiveness); lamentation (crying out in distress and asking for vindication); adoration (giving honor and praise); invocation (summoning the presence of the Almighty); and thanksgiving (offering gratitude). One person's prayers may employ all of these different forms. During the course of your surgery and recovery, you may find yourself praying in all of these ways.

Directed Versus Nondirected Prayer

A distinction has been made between directed and nondirected prayer. Directed prayer has a specific goal or outcome in mind. In effect, the person praying attempts to "direct" the higher power to intervene in a specific way. For example, one might pray for a specific healing process to occur, or for pain to disappear. Nondirected prayer is an open-ended approach in which no specific outcome is requested. In nondirected prayer, the person does not attempt to "direct" the higher power in any way. A request is simply made that "Thy will be done," with the trust that it will be for the best.

Whether you pray in a directed or nondirected mode depends on your beliefs about a higher power, your situation, or both. As Dr. Dossey points out, for some people highly specific goal-directed prayers seem arrogant as they feel such prayers attempt to tell the higher power what to do. On the other hand, some people prefer a more directed approach. They believe that this helps to ensure that the desired outcome will ultimately result. However, when praying in a directed mode, many people also add the caveat: "If it be Your will." This blends the nondirected and directed approaches.

Intercessory Prayer

Most of the material discussed above focuses on an individual's faith and prayer for his or her own health and recovery. Intercessory prayer is praying for someone else. Praying for others is common in most religions and spiritual belief systems. Those who have faith in the power of prayer know that it works, both for the individual and when praying for others.

Dr. R. Byrd (1988) investigated the efficacy of intercessory prayer using scientific methods. Almost 400 patients who had been hospitalized in a coronary care unit in a San Francisco hospital over a ten-month period were randomly assigned to prayer and control groups. Neither the patients nor their caregivers (doctors, nurses, and other hospital staff) knew who was assigned to which group. Then Dr. Bryd recruited various religious groups to pray for the "prayer" group. No one prayed for the control group. He found that the patients who received the intercessory prayer were five times less likely to need antibiotics and three times less likely to develop pulmonary edema. Also, none of the prayed-for group required endotracheal intubation (an artificial airway placed in the throat) whereas twelve in the control group needed that procedure.

These results are certainly intriguing especially given the fact that the patients did not know they were being prayed for. As Dr. L. Dossey (1993) points out, "If the technique being studied had been a new drug or a surgical procedure instead of prayer, it would almost certainly have been heralded as a 'breakthrough.'" Knowing that others are praying for you when you go through the surgical experience may be of even greater benefit, because you will feel safer, and more connected.

Personality Factors and Prayer

Usually, how a person prays is greatly influenced by his or her personality, for example, whether you are an introvert or extrovert. Generally, introverts are more inner-directed and contemplative and extroverts are more outer-directed and action-oriented. Whether you are more feeling-oriented or thinking-oriented might also influence how you pray.

Action-oriented/extroverted people may equate meditative nondirected prayerfulness with inactivity and surrendering to fate or "giving in." For these personalities, prayer might be a relatively action-oriented process, including praying out loud in groups, taking part in various rituals, and maintaining lengthy prayer lists. Faced with illness and crises, action-oriented people are more likely to be problem-focused. They are also apt to provide "action-packed" advice to others who are going through illness or crises, and they might tend to be more concerned about what the sick person should do, rather than how he or she "should be."

For introverted people, prayer may be very inner-directed, contemplative, and "passive" in the face of crises. For these personalities, prayer is a very personal experience, not to be shared with others. They are more likely to talk about prayer as "listening to God or their Higher Power" and not feel compelled to plan actions, tell others what to do, or testify with their prayers in public spaces such as church.

The importance of these differences in personal styles of prayer is that all of these issues are intensified when facing surgery. For instance, we have worked with people who actually found the support of religious friends and family to be stressful. The following case study illustrates this point:

Michael was preparing for open-heart surgery. It was to be a fairly routine procedure but would require him to stay in the hospital for several days with a rather lengthy rehabilitation period. With his family, Michael had been part of a church for virtually all of his life. Although he was a member of the church, he did not engage in any public aspects of practicing his spiritual beliefs. (He didn't pray in groups, "share" his testimonial, or testify.) He was very religious but also introverted. Thus, he practiced his faith in an introverted manner.

When his family found out he needed the surgery, they activated their church "prayer chain." Michael was happy about this and felt less fearful and more secure knowing that others were praying for him. However, during his recovery, the religious practices of certain action-oriented members of his church became very stress-provoking to him. When they visited him in the hospital, they insisted on praying out loud in a circle around the hospital bed. They would call him on the phone to "pray with him" and also wanted him to pray out loud with them.

This was very stressful for Michael and made him extremely uncomfortable. After much duress, ultimately, he had his wife help him by setting limits on the visits and calls from the action-oriented church members who were pressuring him to pray and worship in their manner.

The important thing to remember throughout your surgery experience is to practice your faith and pray in a manner that is right for you.

The Relaxation Response and Prayer

As described in Chapter 7, the relaxation response "triggers" many positive physiological changes including decreased metabolism, blood pressure, heart rate, rate of breathing, and muscle tension. There may also be further benefits in adding a prayerful component to the relaxation experience. As stated previously, there are many ways to elicit the relaxation response. Dr. Herbert H. Benson's original research involved teaching people to meditate using the word "One," or any other word or phrase with which they were comfortable. They would simply repeat the focus word or phrase over and over while they relaxed their muscles and assumed a passive attitude.

Through the course of his research, Dr. H. Benson observed that a great many of his patients chose a spiritual word or prayer on which to focus. He found, that to his surprise, 80 percent of his patients chose prayers for their focus, regardless of their particular faith.

Ultimately, Dr. H. Benson studied whether choosing a prayer to elicit the relaxation response provided any difference from choosing a secular word. He had some patients use a simple secular focus word, such as *"One, ocean, love, peace,* or *calm."* He had others use religious focus words or prayers. (Examples of these religious phrases can be seen in Table 10.1.)

Table 10.1
Religious Words or Prayers*

Christian (Protestant or Catholic)
> Our Father who art in heaven
> The Lord is my shepherd
> Lord Jesus, help me and protect me
> Blessed be the Lord

Catholic
> Hail, Mary full of grace
> Lord Jesus Christ, have mercy on me

Jewish
> Sh'ma Yisroel
> Jehovah-Shalom (God is my Peace)
> Echod
> Jehovah-Rophe (God is my Healer)

Islamic
> Insha'allah

Hindu/Buddhist
> Om

*Adapted from Dr. Herbert Benson (1996).

Dr. H. Benson found that all of the mantras worked. All were equally effective in stimulating the healthy physiological changes termed "the relaxation response." Interestingly, he also found that those who used the word "One" or similar simple secular phrases did not continue with the program, while those who used prayers and religious phrases did continue.

Dr. H. Benson also discovered that a person's religious convictions or life philosophy enhanced the average effects of the relaxation response in three ways:

1. People who choose an appropriate focus that draws on their deepest philosophical or religious convictions are more apt to stick to the elicitation routine for the relaxation response. They look forward to it and enjoy it.

2. Affirmative beliefs of any kind bring forth brain waves that are associated with wellness.

3. When present, faith in an eternal or life-transcending force seems to make the fullest use of feelings of wellness, because faith has an extremely soothing effect, disconnecting unhealthy worries and anxieties.

In light of Dr. H. Benson's findings, you might find it useful to incorporate a meaningful phrase when you practice eliciting the relaxation response. Using the relaxation techniques from Chapter 7, incorporate your meaningful phrase into your exercise. In the space below, list some meaningful phrases from which you might choose. These phrases can be alternated between your relaxation times and meditation practice.

_____

_____

_____

_____

_____

_____

_____

_____

Do Not Think of Illness as God's Punishment

When working with people who are facing a major surgery, we have found it is not uncommon for the issue of "God's punishment" to arise. People are often reluctant to discuss this feeling initially, but will expand on it extensively once it has been broached. This is the feeling that the illness or trauma that caused the need for surgery occurred because the person is being "punished" by God. Throughout much of recorded history, illness and traumas were believed to be the result of having lost favor with God. This feeling, that somehow the calamity is deserved, can cause a great deal of anger or guilt and interfere significantly with having the best possible response to your surgery.

Managing this type of belief and the guilt that is associated with it is best done by using the cognitive self-talk techniques described in Chapters 5 and 6. The same techniques for stopping, challenging, and reframing can be used for unhealthy spiritual beliefs as well as for any other negative automatic thoughts. To do this, though, one must generate challenging thoughts that are credible.

One way to challenge feelings of guilt and "being punished" is by contemplating both history and your daily newspaper. History is full of examples of bad things happening to good people when there was certainly no reason to think that they deserved it. Consider the children who died during any of this century's wars. They were innocent victims. Or think about the story of Job in the Old Testament, which demonstrates that good people (Job was a "perfect and upright person") can be beset with horrendous experiences. The history books are full of other examples of highly spiritual, God-centered people becoming ill and experiencing a variety of "undeserved" catastrophes. You may have had your own such experiences or know of people for whom this is true.

Alternatively, we can all think of examples in which "bad" people have experienced a continuous stream of fortunate events. In history and current news there are many examples of good things happening to bad people without consequence. These "bad" people have led long and full lives without significant repercussions for their behavior. These facts, considered together, will help you to challenge the idea that health problems and illness always imply a spiritual shortcoming or are a punishment from God. Challenging these beliefs is especially important when you are facing surgery.

In the space below, complete the exercise for negative, unhealthy spiritual thoughts and healthy spiritual thoughts and beliefs. If you have trouble generating healthy spiritual thoughts, consult some of the resources listed in the back of this book, a close friend or family member, or a religious counselor.

Unhealthy Spiritual Thought or Belief   **Healthy Spiritual Thought or Belief**

_____

_____

_____

_____

_____

_____

Case Example: Putting It All Together

Dr. H. Benson (1996), in his book *Timeless Healing,* presents an excellent case study of how to incorporate spirituality into preparing for and recovering from surgery:

> Ann was a thirty-five-year-old admitting clerk who required surgery for a blood clot in her leg. She previously had a very negative experience with anesthesia during a prior surgery and was very anxious about her approaching procedure. As a result, she saw the Reverend Dr. Edmond Babinsky for assistance. In explaining her feelings she stated she "just couldn't face the idea of the operation." Knowing that she was Catholic, Dr. Babinsky explained the relaxation response to her and he printed the instructions for eliciting the response on a laminated card. He also gave her a "meditation stone" (a simple white pebble from the beach).
>
> Ann went smoothly through the surgery. She reported that she was able to elicit the relaxation response and meditate on the phrase "Be still my soul." She would also hold the meditation stone the chaplain had given her, which gave her a sense of comfort and security.

This example demonstrates how spirituality helps one to cope with surgery. It describes how to combine techniques such as the deep relaxation response, cue-controlled relaxation (using the stone as the cue), and prayer to deal successfully with the stress of surgery. The ideas and techniques throughout this book can be adapted to create a program that works for you. This program will be different for each person who reads this book.

Developing Your Spiritual Life

You may be inclined to focus on your spiritual life only when you are confronted with a surgery. The following suggestions may help you to activate, reactivate, or enhance your spirituality:

1. Participate regularly in a spiritual/religious organization. If that is not possible or not desired, having some type of connection with such a group may still be helpful.

2. Read spiritual and inspirational literature frequently on a regular basis.

3. Practice the relaxation response using a prayer as your focus word on a regular basis.

4. Develop affirmations of a spiritual nature to keep with you at all times and review them on a regular basis.

PART V

Taking Control of Your Environment

Part V helps you to take the initiative in making your passage through the medical environment, and the process of surgery and recovery, a positive and efficient experience.

Chapter 11 offers you tools for managing your time through:

- Setting priorities

- Delegating responsibilities

- Allowing extra time in your schedule

- Saying "no" to unwanted demands

- Overcoming procrastination through rewards

Chapter 12 provides skills for positive communication with doctors, medical staff, family, and friends through an assertive, rather than submissive or aggressive, attitude, and through a firm belief in your personal rights.

11

Time Management: Taking Control of Your Time

Time is one of our most valuable resources—in fact, it is the one resource that is not renewable. In the face of such sobering facts, it is ironic that most people feel they cannot take control of their time. They believe they are governed by outside forces such as the need to work overtime to get ahead, the demands of the family, the need to meet other obligations, or just to watch TV. (As an interesting exercise, add up the total number of hours you watch television during the week!)

Time management will help you take control of your time so that you can complete the preparation for surgery program successfully. This is probably the most important aspect of your training, because without it the program will fail. Reading the information in this book is an important first step, but, if the exercises are not practiced regularly, it will do no good. It is like buying the best touring bicycle available with the intent of learning how to ride. If you don't practice and acquire the skill, you might just as well have purchased a tricycle.

Time management enables you to set aside enough time to practice the relaxation exercises and other procedures in this guidebook. It can also improve the overall quality of your life. The most important thing to remember as you apply these exercises is *how you spend your time is your choice!*

Time Out

Time out is time you set aside for yourself away from responsibilities such as work, obligations, and chores. Time out can be spent in several ways, such as rest time, recreation time, and relationship time.

Rest time is achieved by setting aside all activities and allowing yourself just to be passive or immersing yourself in something you enjoy. It might be meditating, listening to music, or taking a nap. It is productive not according to societal standards (at least in our Western culture) but rather for yourself.

Recreation time is time set aside for planned activities that you enjoy. These activities are fun and playful, and "recreate" you.

Relationship time is time spent with another person, or other persons, to enjoy the interaction and to maintain or build the intimacy of the relationship(s).

These three types of Time Out are all necessary for a sense of personal self-fulfillment. They are also necessary parts of a surgery preparation program, both before and after your operation. Unfortunately, it is just this kind of time that is likely to be neglected as the stress of the surgery and recovery process comes bearing down. It is important to note that, depending on your medical condition and the type of surgery you are having, you may need to adjust the types of Time Out you give yourself. In any case, Time Out is important for everyone and can be developed no matter what your physical condition might be.

In the following spaces record how you make use of each of the three types of Time Out. Then, assess whether your use of Time Out is adequate or needs improvement. After that, record how you might make the time for specific activities under the three types of Time Out. In completing this task, it is useful to get feedback from others who are close to you. Often we are unrealistic when it comes to assessing our own Time Out (e.g., the businessperson who works eighty hours per week, has multiple stress-related illnesses, plays golf once a week with business contacts, and feels that "everything is fine").

Time Out Activity	*Adequate or Improve?*	*Strategy to Change*
Rest Time		

_____

_____

_____

_____

_____

Recreation Time

_____

_____

_____

_____

_____

Relationship Time

_____

_____

_____

_____

_____

Setting Priorities

Prioritizing means determining the relative importance of various activities. This determination will often change as certain activities move to the top of the list and others move off the list. In setting priorities, it can be useful to categorize activities as essential, important, and trivial. Essential activities are those that require immediate attention and must be completed. Important tasks need to be completed but may not require immediate attention. Last, trivial tasks are those that can be postponed, delegated to others, or declined altogether.

In order to get the most out of the surgery preparation program, most of the exercises must be placed in the essential category. To help you do this, think of the program in terms of taking care of yourself. Remember, time is your most important resource, and the techniques in this book are aimed at giving you more quality time to do the things you enjoy by:

- Decreasing anxiety and tension before the surgery and providing emotional and physical calm

- Improving the quality of your time as you go through the process of surgery and recovery

- Decreasing the amount of time needed to recover from your surgery

- Improving your overall outcome

There is a weekly prioritization chart at the end of this chapter. Copy this chart and use it on a weekly basis to ensure that the tasks related to your surgery management program are completed.

Delegating

Delegating is having someone else take care of a task for you. There can be several reasons for delegating activities, such as having too many responsibilities already, keeping your stress level down, or knowing that a specific activity might be better handled by another person with skills in that area. Delegating responsibility to others can free you from overloading yourself with too many activities. It is important to remember that when delegating responsibility you may need to let go of some control and relax your standards. Others may not do a task exactly as you would, but when you are in need they can still get it done adequately.

Delegating some responsibilities related to your surgery can be extremely helpful. Of course, there are certain things only you can do (i.e., going to doctor's appointments and completing most of the exercises in this book). Even so, there are many other ancillary tasks related to your surgery that can be delegated to others. Here are a few examples:

- Have someone help you complete the medical fact sheet in Chapter 2 by asking you questions about your history.

- Have a significant other help you gather past medical records.

- Have someone organize distracting activities in your home for use during your postoperative recovery and rehabilitation. This might include getting together a number of books you want to read, making sure the TV and VCR are working, and setting up the area in your home where you will be spending most of your time.

- Delegate the "traffic management" of your friends, acquaintances, and family members. A significant other can act as gatekeeper for the social visits and involvement of extended family members. This can be important since family members and acquaintances, while well-meaning, can easily cause increased stress with too many questions, unwanted suggestions, and overextended visits.

Have someone get your prescriptions, drive you to appointments, prepare your meals, and take care of errands such as paying bills.

In some situations there is simply no social support available for the delegation of tasks. In this situation you will have to use other time management techniques to take care of the "essential" priorities. You may often be able, with a bit of brainstorming, to find someone to help you. You may think, "Well, my friend, John, could help me with some things but I would hate to ask." Consider your friends, think about reasonable requests (delegation), and ASK!

Allowing Extra Time

It is important to allow adequate time to complete the specific tasks related to the surgery preparation program. In most cases, since this program is used with elective surgeries, time is available prior to the surgery. Even if the time before surgery is short, a realistic amount of time for each specific exercise must be set aside. Be aware of some common time-allocation problems. For example, in doing the relaxation exercise part of the program, you may set aside only ten minutes for an exercise requiring fifteen or twenty minutes or try to "grab" some relaxation exercise time during the course of the day. These approaches will sabotage the exercise and make it ineffective. Allow what may seem like "extra time" to ensure success.

Allow extra time for other activities related to your surgery such as doctor's appointments (and the commute to and from), blood collections, medical tests, or any other procedure for which you may be required to wait. Bring a book to read to calm your frustration while waiting.

Saying "No"

Saying "No" is an essential time-management skill that will enable you to protect yourself against unwanted incursions on your time. It is a valuable skill not only for surgery management but for all aspects of life. We will focus more extensively on saying "no" without feeling guilty in Chapter 12.

Procrastination

Procrastination is self-defeating. There are two common reasons for procrastination: You may not want to do what needs to be done, or you strive for perfection. In the first case, the key to overcoming procrastination is in prioritizing or delegating. Delegating the task will solve the problem immediately. Prioritizing still makes it incumbent upon you to complete a task, but it does put it *on the list*. One way to overcome procrastination is to develop a reward for completing the task that is being put off. Make a contract with yourself, or with someone else, that once you complete the task you will obtain the reward. Consider the following example:

> Steve was having trouble prioritizing his relaxation exercises. He would practice "when he had time." This "time" seemed to be rare! To increase his compliance with the exercises we started a reward system. It was agreed that he would receive a small reward if he did the assigned practice for the day and then a more substantial reward if he completed the exercises for the week. Steve greatly enjoyed his time playing with computer programs or watching educational TV. Therefore, these activities were chosen as daily rewards. If the relaxation exercises were completed he was allowed his computer or TV time. Otherwise, it was withheld. A weekly reward was also established. This program worked so well that after a while the relaxation exercises became a reward in and of themselves, and external rewards were no longer needed.

This example illustrates several important points about reinforcers.

First, decide on the target behavior and define it very specifically so that there is no doubt about its actual completion. As an example, relaxation could be defined as "taking it easy for a little while at least once a day" or "practicing the relaxation exercises once a day." In the first case there is a high degree of discretion as to whether the task was completed or not. In the second case, there is no question.

Second, choose reinforcers that are actually rewarding. A reinforcer can be anything that increases the frequency of a desired behavior, and may be specific to the individual. For one person a bowl of fresh spinach may be a powerful reinforcer and for another it may be a punishment. A reward should be something you want to do, or have, so much so that you are willing to engage in your target behavior (i.e., the relaxation exercise) to obtain it.

Third, a reward should be something that is easily dispensed, within your immediate control, and nonstressful. For instance, a new car might be a great reward, but the monthly car payments may not be. In setting up your reward program, *be realistic.*

Fourth, follow two important rules: Don't cheat and give yourself the reward without earning it, and be sure to give yourself the reward when you do earn it.

Fifth, if possible, have someone else help to monitor your reward contract with yourself. This creates "accountability" and can dramatically increase your compliance.

In the spaces below, fill in your short-term and long-term rewards and the behaviors you think you might need to reinforce. These tasks can even be single events such as, "Once I complete this medical test, which I don't want to do, I will get . . ." You can return to this table at any time and add activities as you become aware of procrastination.

Rewards for Completing Tasks

Task	*Short-Term Reward (if applicable)*	*Long-Term Reward*
Relaxation exercise twice per day	Computer/TV in evening	if done 5 out of 7 days purchase new book

Priority Log for the Week of _____ *

Use this log to establish priorities for each week. After each priority, circle whether it is essential, important, or trivial. During the week, you can then focus your attention accordingly.

Priority	Category		
_____	Essential	Important	Trivial
_____	Essential	Important	Trivial
_____	Essential	Important	Trivial
_____	Essential	Important	Trivial
_____	Essential	Important	Trivial
_____	Essential	Important	Trivial
_____	Essential	Important	Trivial
_____	Essential	Important	Trivial
_____	Essential	Important	Trivial
_____	Essential	Important	Trivial
_____	Essential	Important	Trivial
_____	Essential	Important	Trivial
_____	Essential	Important	Trivial
_____	Essential	Important	Trivial
_____	Essential	Important	Trivial
_____	Essential	Important	Trivial
_____	Essential	Important	Trivial
_____	Essential	Important	Trivial
_____	Essential	Important	Trivial

*You may copy this sheet for weekly use.

12

Working with Your Doctor, Family, and Friends

The process of surgery and postoperative recovery can bring up stressful situations related to working with your doctor, your family, and your friends, in addition to the stress of the surgery itself. Being able to manage these situations effectively is important in enhancing your experience with surgery.

This chapter teaches you to communicate effectively with your doctor, and with your family and friends, to make sure they are actually supportive rather than a source of additional stress. This chapter will discuss communication styles, learning to be assertive, working effectively with your doctor, and interacting in a healthy manner with your family and friends.

Communication Styles

There are four types of communication or behavior styles:

Nonassertive, or *submissive*, behavior is characterized by giving in to another person's preferences while discounting your own rights and needs. When you do this, the people around you may not even be aware that you are being nonassertive or submissive because your needs are never expressed. Nonassertive or submissive behavior may cause you to feel guilty, or resentful that your rights are somehow being "violated," even though, in reality, your needs are never expressed. The fantasy associated with this behavior is that other people "should know" what you want and should respect those feelings. People who are chronically nonassertive often feel the need to please others around them and are afraid they will not be liked if they actually express their desires.

The Doctor-Patient Communication Gap

Although surveys generally show that most Americans are satisfied with their doctors, a significant communication gap appears to exist. For instance, in a recent survey of consumers by the American Medical Association, only 42 percent felt that doctors usually explained things well to their patients and only 31 percent believed that physicians spent enough time with their patients. In addition, the vast majority of complaints to health maintenance organizations involve the manner in which the medical staff communicated with patients (Ferguson 1993).

It has also been found that the average amount of time a general practitioner spends with a patient is only seven minutes. Further, one study found that most doctors interrupt their patients within the first eighteen seconds of their explanation of symptoms. Patients' complaints about doctor-patient communication most commonly include (beginning with the most frequent):

- the doctor not spending enough time with them

- not being friendly

- not answering questions openly

- not explaining problems understandably

- not treating them respectfully

Learning how to communicate with your doctor while preserving the quality of the relationship is essential. The skills discussed in this chapter will help you to accomplish this goal.

The second style is *aggressive* communication, in which you express your wants and desires in a hostile or attacking manner. Typically, aggressive people are insensitive to the rights and feelings of others around them and may use coercion and intimidation to get what they want. People who are the targets of aggressive communication will respond either by withdrawing from the aggressive person, or by becoming defensive and fighting back in a nonyielding manner. Aggressive communications increase the conflict in any situation.

Aggressive behavior can disrupt your program for surgery and recovery. Aggressive demands on your doctor, nurses, and social support network can lead them to withdraw from you or to counterattack in a similarly aggressive manner. Either situation is not healthy. Consider the following example:

Jody was preparing for her abdominal surgery. When interacting with her surgeon's office staff, she would often become quite aggressive, continually making demands and threatening to complain to the doctor about their inadequate performance and "incompetence." Her aggressive behavior toward the nurses and support personnel continued through her hospital stay. Although some of her complaints were not without some basis, she would express these in an assaultive manner. During her hospital stay, the nurses spent less and less time interacting with her and responded more and more slowly to her requests. Upon her discharge from the hospital, she continued her aggressive style when interacting with family members at home. Her family began to spend less and less time at home where she was recovering, which caused Jody to increase her aggressiveness and complaints even more. Throughout the entire course of surgery and recovery, Jody expressed her feelings that the entire experience "pissed her off."

This example illustrates how aggressive behavior can work against you through the course of your surgery experience. This example also illustrates another type of behavior termed *passive-aggressive* behavior. Passive-aggressive behavior is a way of expressing anger in a passive manner. The nursing staff responded to Jody's assaultive behavior by becoming passive-aggressive. They unconsciously expressed their feelings of anger toward her by responding more slowly to her requests. Some people express all their anger in this passive-aggressive manner. However, expressing anger in this way is very ineffective communication and often will result in your needs not being understood nor met by other people. If you scored high on the anger scale in Chapter 2, be aware of a possible propensity toward communicating aggressively.

Assertive behavior is an alternative to the above styles. Assertive communication is a way of expressing how you feel or what you want while respecting the rights of others. It involves communicating in a simple and direct fashion without attacking, manipulating, or discounting those around you. Communicating in an assertive fashion allows you to express your needs and desires while keeping those around you comfortable and nondefensive. The following example illustrates assertive behavior:

Mark was having trouble getting the information he wanted about his surgery. He had written down five important questions he wanted his doctor to answer before undergoing the procedure. On previous visits, the surgeon had been reassuring but rather brief in her explanations. She would simply respond to Mark's request for information by saying, "Don't worry about it. I've done hundreds of these, and there won't be a problem." On Mark's next visit to the surgeon, he said, "I would appreciate specific answers to these five questions I have written down about my surgery and the recovery." The surgeon began to respond with her usual general statements of reassurance. Mark once again expressed his request in an assertive fashion, saying, "I feel it is important for me to have specific answers to these questions. I would very much appreciate it if you would give me brief answers to each one of my concerns." The surgeon then responded by answering the questions and Mark thanked her for responding to his request.

In this example, Mark used assertive communication to get the answers to his questions. It is important to note that Mark did not attack the surgeon, nor did he stop making his request when she initially responded in her generalizing fashion. If Mark had attacked her aggressively, he might have obtained the information, but future interactions with her may have become tense and nonproductive.

Becoming Assertive

An essential part of becoming assertive is believing that you have certain basic rights. Many people who are submissive, nonassertive, or passive-aggressive have trouble believing in their basic rights as human beings. To deal with this issue, Dr. E. J. Bourne (1995) has developed a "Personal Bill of Rights" which follows:

Personal Bill of Rights

1. I have the right to ask for what I want.

2. I have the right to say "no" to requests or demands I can't meet.

3. I have the right to express all of my feelings, positive or negative.

4. I have the right to change my mind.

5. I have the right to make mistakes and not have to be perfect.

6. I have the right to follow my own values and standards.

7. I have the right to say no to anything when I feel I am not ready, it is unsafe, or it violates my values.

8. I have the right to determine my own priorities.

9. I have the right *not* to be responsible for others' behaviors, actions, feelings, or problems.

10. I have the right to expect honesty from others.

11. I have the right to be angry at someone I love.

12. I have the right to be uniquely myself.

13. I have the right to feel scared and say "I'm afraid."

14. I have the right to say "I don't know."

15. I have the right not to give excuses or reasons for my behavior.

16. I have the right to make decisions based on my feelings.

17. I have the right to my own needs for personal space and time.

18. I have the right to be playful and frivolous.

19. I have the right to be healthier than those around me.

20. I have the right to be in a nonabusive environment.

21. I have the right to make friends and be comfortable around people.

22. I have the right to change and grow.

23. I have the right to have my needs and wants respected by others.

24. I have the right to be treated with dignity and respect.

25. I have the right to be happy.

Review the Personal Bill of Rights on a regular basis. This can help you to believe in your rights and form the foundation for assertive behavior. It can also help you to feel good about being assertive and to effectively communicate your wants and needs.

Assertive Communication

Assertive communication is a skill that can be learned like any other behavior. The following guidelines will help you learn how to make an assertive request.

Use assertive nonverbal behavior. Your body language communicates a great deal beyond what you express verbally. For instance, if you make a request while looking down at the floor, avoiding eye contact, speaking softly, and turning slightly away from the other person, you are not likely to be taken seriously. Assertive behavior includes staying calm, establishing eye contact, maintaining an open posture, and standing straight with your head up.

Keep your request simple. Keep your assertive request simple, direct, and straightforward. Ask for only one thing at a time—a multitude of requests can be confusing. Easy-to-understand sentences such as "I would like more information about my surgery," or "I would like more information about how to obtain a second opinion," are effective and assertive communications.

Be specific. Ascertain what your wants, needs, and feelings are, so that you can express them in a specific way. When you make an assertive request, be specific. For instance, the request, "I would like to get more help from your office staff regarding my surgery" is vague and may be difficult for your doctor to act on. A more effective communication would be, "I would appreciate your office staff

Assert Yourself—Avoid Infection

You would like to believe that hospitals are clean and sterile, and that you are safe from germs while in one. New research suggests that this is simply not true (Griffin 1996).

The chance that you or a loved one will get an infection during a hospital stay is surprisingly high (5 to 10 percent). Each year, more Americans die from hospital infections than from car accidents and homicides combined. The most vulnerable patients are the elderly, immune suppressed, and the very young. To make things worse, some germs are becoming impervious to anything but the most high-powered antibiotics.

It is disturbing to note that many of these hospital-caused infections can be prevented. The Center for Disease Control estimates that one third of all hospital-acquired infections could be prevented if proper infection control rules were followed. One of the most important guidelines of infection control (and most violated) is proper hand washing by the staff. In a review of 37 studies on hand-washing, it was found that doctors and nurses typically wash their hands only 40 percent of the time, even in intensive care units! You can protect yourself by taking the following steps:

1. Stay as healthy as possible prior to the hospitalization and surgery. This will strengthen your immune system to combat germs.

(Continued on following page)

helping me with the following issues regarding my surgery: insurance preapproval, setting up an appointment for my blood donation, and giving me information about pain control." This latter request is specific, direct, and nonaggressive.

2. Make sure that anyone (doctors, nurses, family, friends) who will be touching you washes their hands in your presence. If a hospital worker comes in with gloves, have them remove them, wash, and change to a new pair.

3. Ask that any presurgery antibiotics be given no more than two hours beforehand. This will ensure that the antibiotics peak when the incision is made.

4. Ask how long you'll need a urinary catheter and have it removed as soon as your doctor gives the OK. These are sometimes kept in longer for the convenience of the staff.

5. Get a copy of the hospital's JCAHO report and look at the infection control section (708-916-5600).

6. Call the hospital and find out how many infection control specialists are on staff and how many patients are in the hospital. The recommended rate is one specialist for every 200 patient beds.

7. Call the head of infection control (often a nurse epidemiologist) and ask if he or she is certified by the Certification Board in Infection Control.

Taking any or all of the steps above will require the assertiveness skills you are learning in this chapter. You can be "friendly but firm" to achieve good protection from germs.

Use "I" statements. Assertive communication uses "I" statements. These usually begin with:

I would appreciate it if . . .
I would like to . . .
I need to . . .

It is important to avoid using "You" statements. Statements starting with, *"You* need to help me out more," or *"You* need to be more compassionate," sound threatening and may put the other person on the defensive.

Address your requests to behaviors and not personalities. Address the specific behaviors of another person rather than "personality features." If you want to express that you are having a problem with something a person is doing, be sure to address the behavior and not the person. For instance, you might say, "I would like you to take over the heavy household chores while I am recovering from my surgery." This is preferable to, "I know this is a difficult request because you tend to be careless about housekeeping, but could you help me with the household chores while I am recovering from my surgery?"

Don't apologize for your request. People who tend to be submissive or nonassertive often make requests in an apologetic manner. Because they may be "people pleasers," they believe that any request they make is an imposition on those around them. Therefore, they may make requests in the form of, "I'm really sorry to have to ask, but do you think it would be possible if, maybe, you could help me with preparing for my surgery, just a little?" This type of request has a very low probability of being acknowledged and expresses that the person making the request does not feel deserving or has the right to ask. If you truly accept the Personal Bill of Rights as your own, you will not feel compelled to apologize for making a reasonable request, or to take responsibility for pleasing those around you. When you make a straightforward, assertive request, the other person can simply accept the request or discuss other options.

Make a request, not a demand. Assertive communication may take the form of making a request or of setting a limit by saying, "no." In either case, the communication should always be done in a manner that respects the rights and dignity of the other person.

Learning to Say "No." Learning to say "no" is an important assertive behavior. This skill is essential for setting limits on the demands of family, friends, and work, as you prepare for and recover from your surgery. People who are submissive or nonassertive often have trouble saying "no" because they feel it undermines their desire to please those around them. When they say "no," they feel guilty and worry that others will not like them.

A simple procedure for saying "no" and setting necessary limits follows:

1. Acknowledge the other person's request by repeating it. This can be done by briefly summarizing the request that has been made.

2. Explain your reasons for declining the request in a simple and straightforward manner.

3. Say "no" to the request.

4. If appropriate, you can suggest an alternative plan that might be acceptable both to you and the person making the request.

The following example illustrates how to use this process for saying "no" and setting limits.

> John was scheduled to undergo prostate surgery which would require a one- or two-week postoperative recovery period at home. John was a successful salesperson who generated quite a bit of income for his company. He was often described by his colleagues as a "workaholic." John informed his supervisor that he would be undergoing the surgery, and would require a two-week postoperative recovery period at home. Initially his supervisor was supportive, but began to ask John if he could follow up on some business issues while he was recuperating. These requests started out as small items, but gradually progressed to the point that John essentially would be working at home during the entire time of his postoperative recovery. His employer even asked if he might come into the office one or two days each week to ensure that he did not get behind in servicing his clients.
>
> Ultimately, John had a discussion with his supervisor to set limits on his work schedule after the surgery. John expressed his needs in the following way: "I understand that you would really like me to service these accounts while I am recovering from my surgery at home." (*acknowledgment*) "I have discussed this with my doctor and he feels it would be unhealthy for me to work at all for the two weeks after the surgery." (*explanation*) "Therefore, I will not be able to work on these accounts while I am recovering." (*saying "no"*) "I will be able to alert all my clients that I will be undergoing surgery and that I can address any problems upon my return." (*alternative option*)

Learning to say "no" is very important when dealing with family, friends, and your work situation. Saying "no" can involve a complex issue such as the one in the above example, or it can be as simple as requesting that family members or friends not visit the hospital during certain hours when you are likely to be resting.

The Broken-Record Technique. The broken-record technique can be effective in assertive communications. It simply involves repeatedly making your request or saying "no" until your communication is acknowledged. If you are just learning how to be assertive, you may be likely to make your request once and then "back down" if you encounter any resistance. The broken-record technique is an effective way to make sure that your request or limit-setting is taken seriously. Consider the following example:

> Mary was at home recovering from her complete hysterectomy. She had a large extended family and social support network. Her friends and family were anxious to visit her and "help" her as she recovered from the surgery. A close friend called and suggested that she come by and visit Mary that afternoon. Initially, Mary stated that she was tired and would be resting during the afternoon, as that was the most difficult time of day for her. Her friend persisted, stating that "she would not be a bother" and could simply sit with Mary. Again Mary reiterated that the afternoon would not be a good time and perhaps the following morning would be better. The friend persisted through five more attempts to suggest that she come by that afternoon. Mary effectively used the broken-record technique by continuing to respond that the following morning would be better. Ultimately, the friend acknowledged her request and scheduled her visit for the following morning.

This example illustrates how the broken-record technique can be effective for setting limits. This is an important skill to master, because patients are often "burned out" by the demands family and friends unwittingly place upon them. On the following lines, write down those situations in which you think you might need to use assertiveness skills and how you might use them. Common situations related to surgery include making requests of your doctor, needs that might arise in the hospital, and interactions with family and friends. You can add to this list as you think of other situations. This exercise can help prepare you for these interactions in advance so that you are not "taken by surprise." And remember, you have the right to change your mind if you decide the arrangements you made are not in your best interest or need to be renegotiated.

Situation   *How You Will Respond Assertively*

_____

_____

_____

_____

_____

_____

_____

Summary of Assertiveness Behaviors

The following is a quick reference summary of assertive communication

- Use assertive nonverbal behavior

- Keep your request simple

- Be specific

- Use "I" statements

- Address your requests to behaviors, not personalities

- Don't apologize for your request

- Make a request, not a demand

- Learn to say "no"

- Use the broken-record technique

Working with Your Doctor

It is essential to have a good working relationship with your doctor. As Dr. H. Benson (1996) points out, "No matter how precise the surgery, studies show you'll recover more quickly if your surgeon is upbeat, confident, and kind." If you trust your physician (review your results on the Trust in Physician Scale from Chapter 1), you can comfortably become an active participant in your medical care. A key part of becoming an active participant is establishing good communications with your doctor. This will help you to express information about your symptoms and concerns effectively, and to get information that you need, while maintaining a positive relationship with your physician. Dr. T. Ferguson (1993) has written extensively in this area, and the following steps have been adapted from his recommendations for improving the quality of doctor-patient communications.

Plan your interview in advance. Before you see your doctor, think about what you would like to accomplish on a particular visit. Make a list of your questions and concerns in a simple and straightforward format. Be realistic about the number of questions that you plan to ask on any given visit. Typically, asking about five questions will allow adequate time for

You Also Are Responsible for Good Communication

You also play a role in good communication with your doctor. Drs. Sherrie Kaplan and Sheldon Greenfield (1989) have determined that the average patient asks fewer than four questions in a fifteen-minute visit with the doctor and one question frequently asked is, "Will you validate my parking?"

Researchers have tried to improve patient communications by coaching patients with chronic illnesses such as diabetes, rheumatoid arthritis, and high blood pressure. The studies involved spending a twenty-minute coaching session with patients prior to their doctor visit. The coaches reviewed the patient's medical chart and helped them generate questions to ask the doctor.

Results showed that the coached patients came away from their visits better satisfied than the uncoached group. The coached group also experienced fewer illness-related limitations to their lifestyles than the uncoached group. For instance, the coached diabetes group had lower follow-up glucose levels, a sign of better diabetes control (Ferguson 1993).

As discussed in Chapter 3, being more assertive with your doctor can result in the patient getting more information but also *decreased* satisfaction with the visit. The manner in which you are assertive with your doctor as well as his or her attitude about the patient role (passive versus active) is probably what determines the quality of the interaction.

discussion. Write the questions down and bring them with you to ensure that you get the information you want. You may also fax your questions to the doctor's office prior to the visit so that they are placed in the medical chart where the doctor can review them just before your visit.

Be assertive. Using the assertiveness skills discussed previously will help you communicate effectively with your doctor and get the information you need. Be assertive, but not aggressive, not only about asking questions, but also in describing your goals for the visit. Doing this at the outset can help the visit go smoothly. For instance, you may start out by telling your doctor that you have five questions or concerns that you would like to get information about.

Check your attitude. Be aware of your attitude when going into the visit with your doctor as your feelings can greatly affect the outcome. For instance, if you are in pain or feeling angry toward doctors, you are likely to be aggressive. The doctor may respond to this aggressiveness with either defensiveness or counteraggressiveness. Either situation does not lead to a pleasant and productive visit.

Let the doctor ask questions first. Your doctor will need to gather a lot of information in a relatively short period of time. Let your doctor ask questions first, then ask for any information that has not been covered or is not clear to you.

Make sure you understand what you and your doctor have concluded. Summarize what you and your doctor have concluded at the end of the visit. If you are uncertain about any instructions or guidelines, address these before you leave. Taking notes during the office visit can be helpful, but don't let it distract you from paying attention to what you doctor is saying.

Direct your questions to the appropriate person. Many surgeons have a physician's assistant or nurse who works closely with him or her. Often, this person can be one of your best sources of additional information about your surgery. Your doctor can also direct you to the office or hospital personnel who can provide the information you want.

Summary of Working with Your Doctor

The following is a brief summary of effective techniques for working with your doctor.

- Plan your interview and visits in advance

- Be assertive

- Check your attitude

- Let the doctor ask questions first

- Make sure you understand what you and your doctor have concluded

- Bring a friend to your doctor visits

- Direct your questions to the appropriate person

Family and Friends

Be assertive with family and friends. Often, family and friends don't know how to act toward a person who is preparing for or recovering from a surgery. In our clinical experience, they may tend towards one of two extremes: either offering too much support, resulting in you being "burned out," or withdrawing to the point of not being available or helpful.

Your assertive communication can help give your family and friends exact information about your needs. These can include such matters as transportation to and from doctor's visits, helping you gather information, taking over certain responsibilities while you are recovering from the surgery, and setting limits on visiting and socializing.

In the space below, write down what you would like your family and friends to help you with before surgery, while you are in the hospital, and during your recovery. Also record how you might need to set limits (e.g., visiting times, making demands on you while you are recovering, etc.)

Take a Friend to Your Visit With the Doctor

One of the most effective methods for getting the most out of your visit with the doctor is to bring a friend or family member with you. This is especially true if you are facing an important medical decision or gathering information from a specialist.

Dr. T. Ferguson (1993) concludes that bringing another person with you can help in many ways. Some of these ways are as follows:

- Your friend's presence helps keep you calm and relaxed so that you can focus better

- With someone else along, you are less likely to feel intimidated.

- Your companion can bring up questions or concerns and help you recall what was discussed with the doctor

- Your friend can act as a "reality check" on how the visit with the doctor went

It can also be helpful to develop a strategy with your friend or family member before the visit with the doctor. This might include jointly using the techniques suggested in this chapter.

Before Surgery

_____

_____

_____

_____

_____

During the Hospitalization

_____

_____

_____

_____

_____

After the Surgery

_____

_____

_____

_____

_____

Appendices

This workbook was designed to help you establish an individualized preparation and recovery from surgery program. These Appendices are provided to help you find specific information about your surgery and related issues. Further information can be obtained from the References and Resources Section and from the following directories:

Backus, K., ed. 1993. *Medical and Health Information Directory: Vol 1. Organizations, Agencies, and Institutions*, 6th ed. Detroit, MI: Gale Research.

Daniels, P. K., and C. A. Schwartz, eds. 1994. "Health and medical organizations." In *Encyclopedia of Associations: Vol. 1 Part 2: National organizations of the U.S.*, 28th ed., pp. 1415-1700. Detroit, MI: Gale Research.

Appendix A

Organizations Specific to
Disease and Health

AIDS

Centers for Disease Control
National AIDS Hot Line
800/342-AIDS (342-2437)

National Association of People with AIDS
800/HIV-INFO (448-4636)

Asthma and Allergy

Allergy Control Products
96 Danbury Road
Ridgefield, CT 06887
800/422-DUST (422-3878)

Allergy Foundation of America
801 Second Avenue
New York, NY 10017
212/684-7875

American Academy of Allergy and
  Immunology
611 East Wells Street
Milwaukee, WI 53202
800/822-2762

American College of Allergy and
  Immunology
85 West Algonquin, Suite 550
Arlington Heights, IL 60005
800/842-7777

Asthma and Allergy Foundation of America
1717 Massachusetts Avenue NW, Suite 305
Washington, DC 20036
202/265-0265

Asthma Information Center
P.O. Box 790
Springhouse, PA 19477-0790
800/727-5400

Canadian Society of Allergy and Clinical
    Immunology
Victoria General Hospital
P.O. Box 5375
800 Commissioner's Road East
London, Ontario N6A 4G5
519/685-8167

Alzhiemer's Disease

Alzhiemer's Association
919 North Michigan Ave, Suite 1000
Chicago, IL 60611-1676
800/572-6037

Arthritis

Arthritis Foundation
P.O. Box 19000
Atlanta, GA 30326
404/872-7100
800/283-7800

Back and Spine

National Spinal Cord Injury Association
600 West Cummings Park, Suite 2000
Woburn, MA 01801
800/962-9629

North American Spine Society
6300 N. River Road, Suite 500
Rosemont, IL 60018-4231
708/698-1630

Blood

American Association of Blood Banks
8101 Glenbrook Road
Bethesda, MD 2207
301/907-6977
301/215-6480

Council of Community Blood Centers
725 15th Street NW, Suite 700
Washington, DC 20005
202/393-5725

Department of Health and Human Services
Public Health Service
Food and Drug Administration
Office of Public Affairs
5600 Fishers Lane
Rockville, MD 20857
301/443-3170

Foundation for Blood Research
Scarborough, ME
207/883-4131

National Blood Resources Education Program
Information Center
4733 Bethesda Avenue, Suite 530
Bethesda, MD 20814

National Hemophilia Foundation
1101 17th Street NW
Washington, DC 20036
202/833-0085

Breast Cancer

American Cancer Society
1599 Clifton Road, NE
Atlanta, GA 30329
800/ACS-2345 (227-2345)

Breast Lump and Cervical Cancer
    Information Hotline
800/4-CANCER(422-6237)

Dana-Farber Cancer Institute
Boston, MA
617/632-2178

Lombardi Cancer Research Center
Comprehensive Breast Center
Georgetown University
Washington, DC
202/687-2104
202/687-2113

My Image After Breast Cancer
6000 Stevenson Avenue, Suite 203
Alexandria, VA 22304
703/461-9616

National Alliance of Breast Cancer
  Organizations
1180 Avenue of the Americas, 2nd Floor
New York, NY 10036
212/719-0154

National Cancer Institute
800/4-CANCER (422-6237)

Breast Implants

Food and Drug Administration
Breast Implant Information Service
Office of Consumer Affairs (HFE-88)
5600 Fishers Lane
Rockville, MD 20857
303/433-5006
800/532-4440

Cancer

American Cancer Society
1599 Clifton Road, NE
Atlanta, GA 30329
800/ACS-2345 (227-2345)

Canadian Association of Nuclear Medicine
1980 Sherbrooke Street West #200
Montreal, Quebec H3H 1E8
514/939-3273

British Columbia Cancer Agency
600 West 10th Avenue
Vancouver, British Columbia V5Z 4E6
604/877-6000 ext. 2367

Cancer Conquerors Foundation
P.O. Box 3444
Fullerton, CA 92634
714/671-3850

Cancervive, Inc.
6500 Wilshire Boulevard, Suite 500
Los Angeles, CA 90048
213/203-9232

City of Hope National Medical Center
1500 East Duarte Road
Duarte, CA 91010-3000
818/359-8111

Fred Hutchinson Cancer Research Center
1124 Columbia
Seattle, WA 98104
206/667-5000

Memorial-Sloan Kettering Cancer Center
1275 York Avenue
New York, NY 10021
212/639-2000

National Cancer Institute
Office of Cancer Communications
800/4-CANCER (422-6237)

National Coalition for Cancer Survivorship
1010 Wayne Avenue, Suite 300
Silver Spring, MD 20910
301/585-2616

Reach to Recovery
American Cancer Society
1599 Clifton Road, NE
Atlanta, GA 30329
800/ACS-2345 (227-2345)

Skin Cancer Foundation
245 5th Avenue, Suite 2402
New York, NY 10016
212/725-5176

John Wayne Cancer Institute
2102 Santa Monica Boulevard
Santa Monica, CA 90404
310/315-6125

Childbirth

American Fertility Society
1209 Montgomery Highway
Birmingham, AL 35216
205/978-5000

Center for the Study of Multiple Births
333 East Superior Street, Suite 476
Chicago, IL 60611
312/266-9093

Childbirth Education Association
612/854-8660

International Cesarean Awareness Network
National Office
P.O. Box 152
Syracuse, NY 13210
717/585-4226

March of Dimes Birth Defects Foundation
1275 Mamaroneck Avenue
White Plains, NY 10605
914/428-7100

National Center for Education
in Maternal and Child Health
38th and R Streets, NW
Washington, DC 20057
202/625-8400

National SIDS Foundation
2 Metro Plaza
8240 Professional Place
Landover, MD 20785
319/322-4870

Public Citizen Publications
2000 P Street NW, Suite 600
Washington, DC 20036
202/833-3000

Substance Abuse Program for Pregnant
Women
202/574-2480

Sudden Infant Death Syndrome Headquarters
10500 Little Patuxent Parkway, Suite 420
Columbia, MD 21044
301/459-3388
800/221-7437

Digestion, Bowel Dysfunction, and Incontinence

American Digestive Diseases Society
7770 Wisconsin Avenue
Bethesda, MD 20814
301/652-9293

American Society for Gastrointestinal
Endoscopy
13 Elm Street
Manchester, MA 01944
508/526-8300

Crohn's and Colitis Foundation of America
386 Park Avenue South
New York, NY 10016-8804
800/343-3637

Help for Incontinent People
Box 544
Union, SC 29379
800/252-3337

International Foundation for Bowel
Dysfunction
P.O. Box 17864
Milwaukee, WI 53217
414/964-1799

National Digestive Diseases Information
Clearinghouse
P.O. Box NDDIC
9000 Rockville Pike
Bethesda, MD 20892
301/654-3810

Society for Surgery of the Alimentary Tract
200 First Street, SW
Rochester, MN 55901
507/284-2870

Eyes

American Academy of Ophthalmology
655 Beach Street
San Francisco, CA 94109
415/561-8500

American Association for Pediatric
  Ophthalmology
P.O. Box 193832
San Francisco, CA 94119
415/561-8505

National Retinitis Pigmentosa Foundation
800/683-5555

National Society to Prevent Blindness
500 East Remington Road
Schaumburg, IL 60173
708/843-2020

Hearing

American Hearing Research Foundation
55 East Washington Street, Suite 2022
Chicago, IL 60602
312/726-9670

American Society for Deaf Children
814 Thayer Avenue
Silver Springs, MD 20910
301/585-5400

American Tinnitus Association
Box 5
Portland, OR 97207
503/248-9985

Better Hearing Institute
Box 1848
Washington, DC 20013
800/424-8576

Deafness Research Foundation
9 East 38th Street
New York, NY 10016
800/535-3323

Hearing is Priceless Campaign
House Ear Institute
2100 West 3rd Street, 5th Floor
Los Angeles, CA 90067
213/483-4431

Meniere's Network
2000 Church Street #111
Nashville, TN 32736-0001
615/329-7807

National Hearing Aid Society
20361 Middlebelt
Livonia, MI 48152
800/521-5247

Heart

American College of Cardiology
9111 Old Georgetown Road
Bethesda, MD 20814
301/897-5400

American Heart Association
7272 Granville Avenue
Dallas, TX 75231-4596
214/373-6300
202/822-9380
800/242-8721

Canadian Cardiovascular Society
360 Victoria Avenue #401
Westmount, Quebec H2Z 2N4
514/482-3407

Cardiomyopathy and Transplant Center
Division of Cardiac Surgery
Brigham and Women's Hospital
75 Francis Street
Boston, MA 02115
617/732-7678

Cleveland Clinic
9500 Euclid Avenue
Cleveland, OH 44195
216/444-2200

Congenital Heart Anomalies Support,
Education and Resources
2112 North Wilkins Road
Swanton, OH 43558
419/825-5575

High Blood Pressure Information Center
2121 Wisconsin Avenue NW #410
Washington, DC 20036
202/496-1809

National Institutes of Health
High Blood Pressure Information Center
Bethesda, MD 20892
301/496-1809

Mayo Clinic
200 South West First Street
Rochester, MN 55905
507/284-2511

National Heart, Lung, and Blood Institute
National Institutes of Health
9000 Rockville Pike
Bethesda, MD 20892
301/496-4000
301/496-4236

Society for Cardiac Angiography and
    Intervention
P.O. Box 40279
San Francisco, CA 94150
415/647-1668

Hereditary Diseases

Hereditary Disease Foundation
Columbia University
722 West 168th Street #58
New York, NY 10032-2603
212/960-5650

Hospice

Children's Hospice International
700 Princess Street, Suite 3
Alexandria, VA 22314
703/684-0330
800/242-4453

National Hospice Organization
1901 North Fort Meyer Drive, Suite 307
Arlington, VA 22209
703/243-5900
800/658-8898

Jaw, Dental, and Oral Problems

American Academy of Cosmetic Dentistry
2711 Marshall Court
Madison, WI 53705
608/238-6529
800/543-9220

American Association of Oral and
    Maxillofacial Surgeons
9700 West Bryn Mawr Avenue
Rosemont, IL 60018-5701
708/768-6200
800/822-6637
800/467-5268

American Association of Orthodontists
401 North Lindbergh Boulevard
St. Louis, MO 63141-7816
314/993-1700
800/222-9969

American Dental Hygienists Association
444 North Michigan Avenue, Suite 300
Chicago, IL 60611
312/440-8900

American Dental Association
211 East Chicago Avenue
Chicago, IL 60611
312/440-2862

American Society for Dental Aesthetics
635 Madison Avenue
New York, NY 10022
212/751-3263

Cleft Palate Foundation
1218 Grandview Avenue
Pittsburgh, PA 15211
412/481-1376

International Congress of Oral Implantation
248 Lorraine Avenue, 3rd Floor
Upper Montclair, NJ 07043
201/783-6300

National Institutes of Health
National Institute of Dental Research
Building 31
9000 Rockville Pike
Bethesda, MD 20892
301/496-4261

National Oral Health Information
Clearinghouse
Box NOHIC
9000 Rockville Pike
Bethesda, MD 20892
301/402-7364

Kidneys

American Association of Kidney Patients
1 Davis Boulevard, Suite LL1
Tampa, FL 33606
813/251-0725

American Kidney Fund
8110 Executive Boulevard
Rockville, MD 20852
800/638-8299

National Kidney Foundation
30 East 33rd Street
New York, NY 10016
212/889-2210
800/622-9010

Polycystic Kidney Research Foundation
922 Walnut Street
Kansas City, MO 64106
816/421-1869
800/753-2873

Liver

American Association for the Study of
Liver Disease
6900 Grove Road
Thorofare, NJ 08086
609/848-1000

American Liver Foundation
1425 Pompton Avenue
Cedar Grove, NJ 07009
800/223-0179

Mental Health

American Family Therapy Association
2020 Pennsylvania Avenue NW, Suite 273
Washington, DC 20006
202/994-2776

American Mental Health Counselors
Association
5999 Stevenson Avenue
Alexandria, VA 22304
703/823-9800 ext. 383

American Psychiatric Association
1400 K Street NW
Washington, DC 20005
202/682-6000

American Psychological Association
750 First Street NE
Washington, DC 20002-4242
202/336-5700
202/336-5500

American Psychosomatic Society
7628 Old McLean Village Drive
McLean, VA 22101
703/559-9222

American Schizophrenia Association
900 North Federal Highway, Suite 330
Boca Raton, FL 33432
305/393-6167
800/783-3801

American Sleep Disorders Association
1610 14th Street NW, Suite 300
Rochester, MN 55901
507/287-6006

Canadian Psychiatric Association
237 Argyle Avenue #200
Ottawa, Ontario K2P 1BP
613/234-2815

Depression Awareness, Recognition and
    Treatment Program
The National Institute of Mental Health
5600 Fishers Lane, Room 15C-05
Rockville, MD 20857
 301/443-3170

Information Resources and Inquiries Branch
National Institute of Mental Health
5600 Fishers Lane, Room 15C-05
Rockville, MD 20857
800/421-4211

National Mental Health Association
1021 Prince Street
Alexandria, VA 22314
703/684-7722
800/969-6642

National Mental Health Consumers'
    Association
311 South Juniper Street, Room 902
Philadelphia, PA 19107
215/735-6082
FAX 215/735-2465

Organ Donation and Transplants

American Association of Tissue Banks
1350 Beverly Road
McLean, VA 22101
703/827-9582

American Society for Artificial Internal
    Organs
P.O. Box C
Boca Raton, FL 33429-0468
407/391-8589

American Society of Transplant Surgeons
6900 Grove Road
Thorofare, NJ 08086
609/848-1000

Canadian Transplant Society
Toronto General Hospital
Gerrard Wing 3-538
200 Elizabeth Street
Toronto, Ontario M5G 2C4
416/595-3111

Children's Organ Transplant Association
2501 Cota Drive
Bloomington, IN 47403
812/336-8872

Eye Bank Association of America
1001 Connecticut Avenue NW, Suite 601
Washington, DC 20036-5504
202/775-4999

Eye Donation Hotline
 800/638-1818
In Maryland
301/269-4031

International Society for Heart and Lung
    Transplantation
435 North Michigan Avenue, Suite 1717
Chicago, IL 60611-4067
 312/644-0828

Red Cross Tissue Donation Services
800/272-5287

United Network for Organ Sharing
1100 Boulders Parkway, Suite 500
P.O. Box 13770
Richmond, VA 23225-8770
800/292-9537

Pain

American Academy of Pain Medicine
3600 Sisk Road, #2-D
Modesto, CA 95356
209/545-0754

American Chronic Pain Association
P.O. Box 850
Rockland, CA 95677
916/632-0922

American Pain Society
5700 Old Orchard Road, First Floor
Skokie, IL 60077
708/966-5595

Biofeedback Institute of America
10200 West 44th Avenue, Suite 304
Wheat Ridge, CO 80033-2840
303/420-2902

International Association for the Study of Pain
909 NE 43rd Street, Suite 306
Seattle, WA 98105-6020
206/547-6409

National Chronic Pain Outreach Association
7979 Old Georgetown Road #100
Bethesda, MD 20814
301/652-4948

National Headache Foundation
5252 North Western Avenue
Chicago, IL 60624
312/878-7715
800/843-2256

Paralysis

American Paralysis Association
500 Morris Avenue
Springfield, NJ 07081
203/379-2690
800/225-0292

Skin

American Academy of Dermatology
930 North Meacham Road
Schaumburg, IL 60168-4014
708/330-0230

American Board of Dermatology
Henry Ford Hospital
Detroit, MI 48202
313/871-8739

American Osteopathic Board of Dermatology
25510 Plymouth Road
Redford, MI 48239
313/937-1200

American Society for Dermatologic Surgery
930 North Meacham Road
Schaumburg, IL 60173
708/330-0230
708/330-9830

National Rosacea Society
220 South Cook Street, Suite 201
Barrington, IL 60010
708/382-8971

Smell and Taste

Smell and Taste Treatment and Research
   Foundation
845 North Michigan Avenue, Suite 930 West
Chicago, IL
312/938-1047

Substance Abuse

Al-Anon
Family Group Headquarters
Box 862, Midtown Station
New York, NY 10018
800/344-2666

Alateen
1372 Broadway
New York, NY 10018
212/302-7240

Alcoholics Anonymous (AA)
475 Riverside Drive, 11th Floor
New York, NY 10115
212/870-3440

Adult Children of Alcoholics (ACA)
World Services Office
2225 Sepulveda Boulevard #200
Torrance, CA 90505
310/534-1815

Children of Alcoholics Foundation
P.O. Box 4185
Grand Central Station
New York, NY 10163-4185
212/754-0656

Cocaine Anonymous
3740 Overland Avenue, Suite H
Los Angeles, CA 90034-6337
800/347-8998

Narcotics Anonymous (NA)
World Service Office
16155 Wyandotte Street
Van Nuys, CA 91406
818/780-3951

National Association of Children of
  Alcoholics (NACOA)
11426 Rockville Park, Suite 100
Rockville, MD 20852
301/468-0985

National Center for Substance Abuse
  Treatment
800/662-4357

National Cocaine Hotline
800/COCAINE (262-2463)

National Council on Alcoholism
800/622-2255

National Institute of Drug Abuse (NIDA)
11426 Rockville Pike
Rockville, MD 20852
310/443-6245
800/662-4357

Substance Abuse Program for Pregnant
  Women
202/754-2480

Weight and Eating Problems

American Anorexia and Bulimia Association
  (AABA)
418 East 76th Street
New York, NY 10021
212/734-1114

American Dietetic Association
P.O. Box 39101
Chicago, IL 60639
800/366-1655

Anorexics/Bulimics Anonymous (ABA)
P.O. Box 112214
San Diego, CA 92111
619/685-3344

Center for the Study of Anorexia and Bulimia
1 West 91st Street
New York, NY 10024
212/595-3449

Food and Drug Administration
5600 Fishers Lane (HFE-88)
Rockville, MD 20857

Foundation for Education About Eating
  Disorders
P.O. Box 16375
Baltimore, MD 21210
410/467-0603

The Image Foundation
P.O. Box 3630
Chicago, IL 60664
312/670-8404

National Anorexic Aid Society
1925 East Dublin Granville Road
Columbus, OH 43229
614/436-1112

National Association of Anorexia Nervosa
  and Associated Disorders
P.O. Box 7
Highland Park, IL 60035
708/831-3438

Appendix B

Professional Societies

Physicians, Surgeons, and Psychologists

American Academy of Cosmetic Surgery
401 North Michigan Avenue
Chicago, IL 60611
312/527-6713
800/221-9808

American Academy of Facial Plastic and
   Reconstructive Surgery
1110 Vermont Avenue NW, Suite 220
Washington, DC 20005-3522
800/332-3223

American Academy of Family Physicians
8880 Ward Parkway
Kansas City, MO 64114
816/333-9700

American Academy of Health Psychology
2100 E. Broadway, Suite 313
Columbia, MO 65201-6082
573/875-1267

American Academy of Orthopaedic Surgeons
6300 North River Road
Rosemont, IL 60018
800/824-BONE (824-2663)

American Academy of Otolaryngology
Head and Neck Surgery
One Prince Street
Alexandria, VA 22314
703/836-4444

American Academy of Pain Management
3600 Sisk Road, #2-D
Modesto, CA 95356
209/545-0754

American Academy of Pain Medicine
5700 Old Orchard Road
Skokie, IL 60077
708/966-9510

American Academy of Physical Medicine and
    Rehabilitation
122 South Michigan Avenue, Suite 300
Chicago, IL 60603
312/922-9633

American Association for Thoracic Surgery
13 Elm Street
Nanchester, MA 01944
508/526-8330

American Association for Women
    Radiologists
1891 Preston White Drive
Reston, VA 22091
703/648-8939

American Association of Hand Surgery
435 North Michigan Avenue, Suite 1717
Chicago, IL 60611
312/644-0828

American Association of Immunologists
9650 Rockville Pike
Bethesda, MD 20814
310/530-7178

American Association of Neurological
    Surgeons
22 South Washington Street
Park Ridge, IL 60068
708/692-9500

American Association of Plastic Surgeons
2317 Seminole Road
Atlantic Beach, FL 32233-5952
904/359-3759

American Association of Plastic Surgery
10666 North Torrey Pines Road
La Jolla, CA 92037
619/554-9940

American Board of Anesthesiology
100 Constitution Plaza
Hartford, CT 06103
203/522-9857

American Board of Emergency Medicine
200 Woodland Pass, Suite D
East Lansing, MI 48823
517/332-4800

American Board of Family Practice
2228 Young Drive
Lexington, KY 40505
606/269-5626

American Board of Medical Specialties
1007 Church Street, Suite 404
Evanston, IL 60210-5913
708/491-9091

American Board of Neurological Surgery
Smith Tower, Suite 2139
6550 Fannin Street
Houston, TX 77030-2701
713/790-6015

American Board of Nuclear Medicine
900 Veteran Avenue, Room 12-200
Los Angeles, CA 90024-1786
310/825-6787

American Board of Obstetrics & Gynecology
4225 Roosevelt Way NE, Suite 305
Seattle, WA 98105
206/547-4884

American Board of Orthopedic Surgery
737 North Michigan Avenue, Suite 1150
Chicago, IL 60611
312/664-9444

American Board of Otolaryngology
5615 Kirby Drive, Suite 936
Houston, TX 77005
713/528-6200

American Board of Plastic Surgery
Seven Penn Center 400
1635 Market Street
Philadelphia, PA 19103
215/587-9322

American Board of Professional Psychology
2100 E. Broadway, Suite 313
Columbia, MO 65201-6082
573/875-1267

American Board of Radiology
300 Park, Suite 440
Birmingham, MI 48009
313/645-0600
313/643-0300

American Board of Surgery
1617 John F. Kennedy Boulevard, Suite 860
Philadelphia, PA 19103-1847
215/568-4000

American Board of Thoracic Surgery
One Rotary Center, Suite 803
Evanston, IL 60210
708/475-1520

American Board of Urology
31700 Telegraph Road, Suite 150
Birmingham, MI 48010
313/646-9720

American Chiropractic Association
1701 Clarendon Boulevard
Arlington, VA 22209
703/276-8800

American Cleft Palate—Craniofacial
   Association
1218 Grandview Avenue
Pittsburgh, PA 15211
412/481-1376

American College of Cardiology
800/888-8823

American College of General Practitioners in
   Osteopathic Medicine and Surgery
330 East Algonquin Road
Arlington Heights, IL 60005
708/228-6090
800/323-0790

American College of Obstetricians &
   Gynecologists
409 12th Street NW
Washington, DC 20024
202/638-5577

American College of Physicians
Independence Mall West
Sixth at Race
Philadelphia, PA 19106-1572
215/351-2400

American College of Radiology
1891 Preston White Drive
Reston, VA 22091
703/648-8902

American College of Radiology
Mammography Accreditation Program
1891 Preston White Drive
Reston, VA 22091
703/648-8900

American College of Rheumatology
60 Executive Park South, Suite 150
Atlanta, GA 30329
404/633-3777

American College of Sports Medicine
401 West Michigan Street
Indianapolis, IN 46202
317/637-9200

American College of Surgeons
55 East Erie Street
Chicago, IL 60611-2797
312/664-4050
312/664-4056

American Federation of Medical
   Accreditation
522 Rossmore Drive
Las Vegas, NV 89110
702/385-6886

American Medical Association
515 North State Street
Chicago, IL 60610
312/464-5000
800/621-8335

American Medical Women's Association
801 North Fairfax, Suite 400
Alexandria, VA 22314
703/838-0500

American Orthopedic Society for Sports
    Medicine
6300 North River Road, Suite 200
Rosemont, IL 60018
708/292-4900

American Osteopathic Board of
    Anesthesiology
17201 East Highway 40, Suite 204
Independence, MO 64055
816/373-4700

American Osteopathic Board of General
    Practice
330 East Algonquin Road, Suite 2
Arlington Heights, IL 60005
708/635-8477

American Osteopathic Board of Internal
    Medicine
5200 South Ellis Avenue
Chicago, IL 60615
312/947-4880

American Osteopathic Board of Obstetrics
    and Gynecology
5200 South Ellis Avenue
Chicago, IL 60615
312/947-4630

American Osteopathic Board of
    Ophthalmology and Otorhinolaryngology
405 Grand Avenue
Dayton, OH 45405
513/222-4213

American Osteopathic Board of Proctology
2815 South Pennsylvania Avenue, Suite 105-A
Lansing, MI 48910
517/484-9885

American Osteopathic Board of Surgery
405 Grand Avenue
Dayton, OH 45405
513/226-2656

American Osteopathic Hospital Association
1454 Duke Street
Alexandria, VA 22314
703/684-7700

American Pain Society
5700 Old Orchard Road, First Floor
Skokie, IL 60077
708/966-5595

American Pediatric Medical Association
800/366-8227

American Psychological Association
750 First Street, NE
Washington, DC 20002-4242
202/336-5700

American Society for Head and Neck Surgery
P.O. Box 41402
Baltimore, MD 21203
410/955-3669

American Society for Laser Medicine and
    Surgery
2404 Stewart Square
Wausua, WI 54401
715/845-9283

American Society for Surgery of the Hand
3025 South Parker Road, Suite 65
Aurora, CO 80014-2911
303/755-4588

American Society of Abdominal Surgeons
675 Main Street
Melrose, MA 02176
617/665-6102

American Society of Anesthesiologists
520 Northwest Highway
Park Ridge, IL 60068-2573
708/825-5586

American Society of Colon and Rectal
  Surgeons
800 East Northwest Highway, Suite 1080
Palatine, IL 60067
708/359-9184

American Society of Contemporary Medicine
  and Surgery
233 East Erie Street
Chicago, IL 60611
312/951-1400

American Society of Maxillofacial Surgeons
444 East Algonquin Road
Arlington Heights, IL 60005
708/228-3327

American Society of Plastic and
  Reconstructive Surgeons
444 East Algonquin Road
Arlington Heights, IL 60005
708/228-9900

Implant Patient Relations
800/635-0635

American Society of Regional Anesthesia
1910 Byrd Avenue
P.O. Box 11086, Suite 100
Richmond, VA 23230-1086
804/282-0010

American Surgical Association
University of North Carolina
Department of Surgery, CB 7245
Chapel Hill, NC 27599-7245
919/966-6320

Association of American Medical Colleges
2450 N Street NW
Washington, DC 20037-1126
202/828-0400

Association of American Physicians and
  Surgeons
1601 North Tucson Boulevard, Suite 9
Tucson, AZ 85716
602/327-4885

Association of Military Surgeons of the US
9320 Old George Road
Bethesda, MD 20814
301/897-8800

Association of University Anesthetists
Department of Anesthesia
University of Washington
Seattle, WA 98121
206/305-3117

Canadian Anesthetists' Society
1 Eglinton Avenue East #209
Toronto, Ontario M4P 3A1
416/480-0602

Canadian Association of General Surgeons
P. O. Box 4730
Edmonton, Alberta T6E 5G6
403/437-1735

Canadian Association of Pediatrics Surgeons
Children's Hospital #AE201
840 Sherbrook Street
Winnipeg, Manitoba R3A 1S1
204/787-4203

Canadian Association of Physical Medicine
  and Rehabilitation
774 Echo Drive, 5th Floor
Ottawa, Ontario K1S 5N8
613/730-6245

Canadian Association of Radiation
  Oncologists
B.C. Cancer Agency
600 West 10th Avenue
Vancouver, British Columbia V5Z 4E6
604/877-6000 ext. 2668

Canadian Association of Radiologists
5101 Buchan Street #510
Montreal, Quebec H4P 2R9
514/738-3111

Canadian Fertility and Andrology Society
774 Echo Drive
Ottawa, Ontario K1S 5NB
613/730-6251

Canadian Neurological Society
906 12th Avenue SW #810
P.O. Box 4220, Station C
Calgary, Alberta T2T 5N1
403/229-9544

Canadian Ophthalmological Society
1525 Carling Avenue #610
Ottawa, Ontario K1Z 8R9
613/729-6779

Canadian Orthopaedic Association
1440 Ste-Catherine Street West #421
Montreal, Quebec H3G 1R8
414/874-9003

Canadian Society for Endoscopic and
   Laparoscopic Surgery
Mount Sinai Hospital
600 University Avenue
Toronto, Ontario M5G 1X5
416/586-3236

Canadian Society for Surgery of the Hand
Toronto Western Division
5 West Wing 3834
399 Bathurst Street
Toronto, Ontario M5T 2S8
416/369-5448

Canadian Society for Vascular Surgery
Victoria Hospital
375 South Street
London, Ontario N6A 4G5
519/667-6780

Canadian Society of Cardiovascular and
   Thoracic Surgeons
University of Alberta Hospital
W.C. MacKenzie Centre #3H2.11
8440 112th Street
Edmonton, Alberta T6G 2B7
403/492-9187

Canadian Society of Colon and Rectal
   Surgeons
2100 Drummond Street #120
Montreal, Quebec H3G 1X1
514/285-1986

Canadian Society of Internal Medicine
774 Echo Drive, 5th Floor
Ottawa, Ontario K1S 5N8
613/730-6244

Canadian Society of Nephrology
Department of Nephrology
St. Michael's Hospital
30 Bond Street
Toronto, Ontario M5B 1W8
416/867-3701

Canadian Society of Otolaryngology—Head
   and Neck Surgery
55 MacGregor Avenue
Toronto, Ontario M6S 2A1
416/760-8190

Canadian Society of Plastic Surgeons
30 St. Joseph Boulevard East #520
Montreal, Quebec H2T 1G9
514/843-5415

Canadian Society of Surgical Oncology
Department of Surgery
St. Paul's Hospital
Comox Building #368
1081 Burrant Street W
Vancouver, British Columbia V6Z 1Y6
604/631-5025

Canadian Thoracic Society
1900 City Park Drive #508
Gloucester, Ontario K1J 1A3
613/747-6776

College of American Pathologists
325 Waukegan Road
Northfield, IL 60093-2750
708/446-8800

Federation of State Medical Boards
of the United States
6000 Western Place #707
Forth Worth, TX 76107
817/735-8445

International Association for the Study of Pain
909 NE 43rd Street, Suite 306
Seattle, WA 98105-6020
206/547-6409

Lipoplasty Society of North America
825 East Golf Road, Suite 1141
Arlington Heights, IL 60005
708/228-9273

National Foundation for Facial
   Reconstruction
317 East 34th Street, Suite 901
New York, NY 10016
212/263-6656
800/422-FACE (442-3223)

Outpatient Ophthalmic Surgery Society
P.O. Box 23220
San Diego, CA 92193
619/692-4426

Royal College of Physicians and Surgeons of
   Canada
774 Promenade Echo Drive
Ottawa, Canada K1S 5NB
613/730-8177
613/730-6212

Royal College of Physicians and Surgeons of
   the USA
16126 East Warren
Detroit, MI 48224
313/882-0641

Royal College of Surgeons
44-71-831-5161 United Kingdom

Second Surgical Opinion Program
Department of Health and Human Services
330 Independence Avenue SW
Washington, DC 20201
202/690-8056
800/638-6833
Maryland
800/492-6603

Society for Vascular Surgery
P.O. Box 850
Hershey, PA 17033
508/526-8330

Society of Cardiovascular Anesthesiologists
P.O. Box 11086
Richmond, VA 23230-1086
804/282-0084

Society of Gynecological Oncologists
   of Canada
Hamilton Regional Cancer Center
699 Concession Street
Hamilton, Ontario L8V 5C2
416/389-5688

Society of Obstetricians and Gynecologists
   of Canada
774 Echo Drive, 5th Floor
Ottawa, Ontario K1S 5N8
613/730-4192

Society of Thoracic Surgeons
11 East Wacher Drive, Suite 600
Chicago, IL 60601

Society of University Surgeons
P.O. Box 7069
New Haven, CT 06519
203/932-0541

Nurses

American Academy of Nurse Practitioners
Capitol Station, LBJ Building
P.O. Box 12846
Austin, TX 78711
512/442-4262

American Association of Critical Care Nurses
101 Columbia
Aliso Viejo, CA 92656
800/899-2226

American Association of Nurse Anesthetists
222 South Prospect Avenue
Park Ridge, IL 60068-4001
708/692-7050

American College of Nurse-Midwives
818 Connecticut Avenue NW, Suite 900
Washington, DC 20006

American Nurses Association
600 Maryland Avenue SW, Suite 100 West
Washington, DC 20024-2571
202/554-4444
800/274-4262

American Nurses Credentialing Center
600 Maryland Avenue SW, Suite 100 West
Washington, DC 20024-2571
800/284-2378

American Psychiatric Nurses' Association
6900 Grove Road
Thorofare, NJ 08086
609/848-7990

American Society of Post-Anesthesia Nurses
11512 Allecingie Parkway, Suite C
Richmond, VA 23235
804/379-5516

American Society of Plastic and
    Reconstructive Surgical Nurses
Box 56, North Woodbury Road
Pitman, NJ 08071
609/589-6247

Association of Women's Health, Obstetric and
Neonatal Nurses
700 14th Street NW, Suite 600
Washington, DC 20005-2019
202/662-1600

National Association of Pediatric Nurse
    Associates and Practitioners
1101 Kings Highway North, Suite 206
Cherry Hill, NJ 08034
609/667-1773

National Black Nurses Association
1660 L Street NW, Suite 907
Washington, DC 20036
202/673-4551

National League of Nursing
350 Hudson Street
New York, NY 10014
212/989-9393

Physician Assistants

American Academy of Physician Assistants
950 North Washington Street
Alexandria, VA 22314
703/836-2272

Prosthetics

American Orthotic and Prosthetic Association
1650 King Street, Suite 500
Alexandria, VA 22314-1885
703/836-7116

Appendix C

Elderly Person's Resource List

Administration on Aging
330 Independence Avenue SW, Room 4284
Washington, DC 20201
202/619-2598

Alzheimer's Association
919 North Michigan Avenue
Suite 1000
Chicago, IL 60611-1676
800/621-0379

American Association of Homes for the Aging
1129 20th Street NW
Washington, DC 20036
202/783-2242
202/296-5960

American Association of Retired Persons
   (AARP)
601 E Street NW
Washington, DC 20049
301/427-9611
202/434-2277

American Healthcare Association
1201 L Street NW
Washington, DC 20005
202/842-4444

Children of Aging Parents
1609 Woodbourne Road
Levittown, PA 19057
215/345-5104

Elderly Support Network
P.O. Box 248
Kendall Park, NJ 08824-0248
800/634-7654

Gray Panthers
1424 16th Street NW
Washington, DC 20036
202/347-6471

National Association of Area Agencies on
 Aging
1112 16th Street
Washington, DC 20036
202/296-8130

National Association of Geriatric Care
 Managers
655 North Alveran Way
Tucson, AZ 85711
602/881-8008

National Association of State Units on Aging
2033 K Street NW
Washington, DC 20006
202/785-0707

National Citizen's Coalition for Nursing
 Home Reform
1224 M Street NW
Washington, DC 20005
 202/393-2018

National Council of Senior Citizens
1331 F Street NW
Washington, DC 20004-1171
202/347-8800

National Council on Aging
Washington, DC
202/497-1200
800/424-9046

National Institute on Aging
P.O. Box 8057
Gaithersburg, MD 20898-8057

National Senior Citizen's Law Project
2025 M Street NW
Washington, DC 20036
202/887-5280
213/482-3550

Social Security Administration
800/772-1213

United Seniors Health Cooperative
1331 H Street NW
Washington, DC 20005
202/393-6222

Widowed Persons Service (of the AARP)
P.O. Box 199
Long Beach, CA 90801
310/427-9611

Appendix D

Organizations Specific to Children's Health

Association of Research on Childhood Cancer
3653 Harlem Road
Buffalo, NY 14215
716/838-4433

Pediatric AIDS Foundation
1311 Colorado Avenue
Santa Monica, CA 90404
310/395-5149

American Academy of Pediatric Dentistry
211 East Chicago Avenue, Suite 1036
Chicago, IL 60611
312/337-2169

American Academy of Pediatrics
141 Northwest Point Boulevard
Elk Grove, IL 60007
708/228-5005
800/433-9016

American Board of Pediatrics
111 Silver Cedar Court
Chapel Hill, NC 27514
919/929-0461

American Pediatric Society
141 Northwest Point Boulevard
Elk Grove, IL 60009-0675
708/426-0205

American Pediatric Surgical Association
750 Terrado Place, Suite 119
Covina, CA 91723-3419
818/915-5884

American Society for Deaf Children
814 Thayer Avenue
Silver Springs, MD 20910
301/585-5400

American Society of Dentistry for Children
211 East Chicago Avenue, Suite 1430
Chicago, IL 60611
312/943-1244

Association for the Care of Children's Health
7910 Woodmont Avenue, Suite 300
Bethesda, MD 20814-3015
301/654-6549

Children in Hospitals, Inc.
31 Wilshire Park
Needham, MA 02192
617/482-2915

Children's Craniofacial Association
10210 North Central Expressway
Suite 230, Lockbox 37
Dallas, TX 75231
214/368-3590

Children's Leukemia Foundation
29777 Telegraph Road Suite 1651
Southfield, MI 48034
810/353-8222
800/825-2536

Children's Liver Foundation
15 Barton Drive
West Orange, NJ 07052
201/761-1111

Cleft Palate Foundation
1218 Grandview Avenue
Pittsburgh, PA 15211
800/242-5388

Federation of Families for Children's Mental
   Health
1021 Prince Street
Alexandria, VA 22314-2971
703/684-7710

Juvenile Diabetes Foundation
432 Park Avenue South
New York, NY 10016
212/889-7575
800/223-1138

National Association of Pediatric Nurse
   Associates and Practitioners
1101 Kings Highway North, Suite 206
Cherry Hill, NJ 08034
609/667-1773

National Center for Education in Maternal
   and Child Health
8201 Greensboro Drive, Suite 600
McLean, VA 22101
703/821-8955

National Children's Eye Care Foundation
32100 Meadowlark Way
Pepper Pike, OH 44124
216/360-0074

National Information Center for Children
   and Youths with Disabilities
 800/695-0285

National Vaccine Information Center
204-F Mill Street
Vienna, VA 22180
703/938-3783

Research Trust for Metabolic Diseases in
   Children/England
Golden Gate Lodge
Weston Road
Crewe, Cheshire CWI IXN England
011-44-1270-0221

Society for Pediatric Research
141 Northwest Point Boulevard
P.O. Box 675
Elk Grove Village, IL 60009
708/427-0205

Appendix E

General Information and Resources

The Agency for Healthcare Policy and
    Research
Executive Office Center, Suite 501
2101 East Jefferson Street
Rockville, MD 20852
800/358-9295

The Center for Medical Consumers
237 Thompson Street
New York, NY 10012-1090
212/674-7105

Common Cause
2030 M Street NW, Suite 300
Washington, DC 20036-3380
202/833-1200

Consumer Product Safety Commission
5401 Westbard Avenue
Bethesda, MD 20892
800/638-2772
800/492-8104

Drug Enforcement Administration
Department of Justice
1405 1st Street NW
Washington, DC 20005
202/401-7834

The Federal Trade Commission
Correspondence Branch
6th Street and Pennsylvania Avenue NW
Washington, DC 20580
202/326-2180

Food and Drug Administration
Consumer Affairs and Information
5600 Fishers Lane, HFC-110
Rockville, MD 20857
301/443-1544

Gray Panthers
1424 16th Street NW
Washington, DC 20036
202/347-6471

Medication Error Report Program
800/233-7767

National Association of Chain Drug Stores
c/o Ronald L. Ziegler
413 North Lee Street
Alexandria, VA 22313-1417
703/549-3001

National Association of Retail Druggists
205 Dangerfield Road
Alexandria, VA 22314
703/683-8200

National Center for Patients Rights
666 Broadway, Suite 410
New York, NY 10012
212/979-6670

National Citizen's Coalition for Nursing
Home Reform
1224 M Street NW, Suite 301
Washington, DC 20005
202/393-2108

National Headquarters—Council of Better
Business Bureau, Inc.
4200 Wilson Boulevard
Arlington, VA 22203
703/276-0100

National Institute of General Medicine
Sciences
Office of Research Reports
Building 31, Room 4A52
Bethesda, MD 20982
301/496-7301

National Institute of Health
5333 Westbard Ave.
Bethesda, MD 20892
301/496-7326
800/352-9424

National Society of Patient Representatives
and Consumer Affairs of the American
Hospital Association
840 North Lake Shore Drive
Chicago, IL 60611
312/280-6424

National Women's Health Network
1325 G Street NW, Lower Level
Washington, DC 20005
202/347-1140

Nonprescription Drug Manufacturers'
Association
1150 Connecticut Avenue NW
Washington, DC 20036
202/429-9260

People's Medical Society
462 Walnut Street
Allentown, PA 18102
215/770-1670

Pharmaceutical Manufacturers' Association
1100 15th Street NW
Washington, DC 20005
202/835-3400

Public Citizen Health Research Group
2000 P Street NW
Washington, DC 20036
202/833-3000

Public Citizen Publications
2000 P Street NW, Suite 600
Washington, DC 20036
202/833-3000

Safe Medicine for Consumers
P.O. Box 878
San Andreas, CA 95249
209/754-4408
FAX 209/736-2402

References and Resources

Introduction

Bradley, E.L. 1994. *A Patient's Guide to Surgery*. New York: Consumer Reports Books.
This book presents valuable information about what to expect before, during, and after surgery. Discussions on how to choose your surgeon, choosing a hospital, and descriptions of common surgical procedures.

Center for Disease Control (CDC) Website (www.cdc.gov).
This is the national resource for health care information. This website contains a wealth of information regarding most health issues. For example, it links to the National Center of Health Statistics, which can provide statistical information on various surgical procedures.

Devine, E.C. 1992. "Effects of Psychoeducation Care for Adult Surgical Patients: A Meta-Analysis of 191 Studies." *Patient Education and Counseling*, 19:129-142.

Huddleston, P. 1996. *Prepare for Surgery, Heal Faster: A Guide of Mind-body Techniques*. Cambridge, MA: Angel River Press.
This book contains information on mind-body techniques for surgical coping. It focuses on spiritual interventions.

Inlander, C.B. 1993. *Good Operations, Bad Operations*. New York: Penguin Books.
This book contains information on risk factors and complications that is valuable in helping you consider surgical options.

Inlander, C.B. and E.D. Weiner. 1993. *Take This Book to the Hospital With You*. Avenel, NJ: Wings Books.
This book is packed with information about your health and finances which make surviving a hospital stay much easier.

Johnston, M. and C. Vogel. 1993. "Benefits of Psychological Preparation for Surgery: A Meta-Analysis." *Annals of Behavoral medicine.* 15(4):245–256.

Macho, J. and G. Cable. 1994. *Everyone's Guide to Outpatient Surgery.* Kansas City, MO: Sommerville House Books.
The advantages and disadvantages to outpatient surgery versus inpatient surgery are discussed. This book also presents questions to ask your doctors, brief descriptions of the most common outpatient surgeries and how to benefit the most from the system.

McCabe, J. (Ingersol, M. ed.) 1994. *Surgery Electives: What to Know Before the Doctor Operates.* Santa Monica, CA: Carmania Books.
Information about the medical profession in general and surgery in particular. The chapters on evaluating doctors, questions to ask and what to expect before, during and after surgery are valuable.

Prokop, C.K., L.A. Bradley, T.G. Burish, K.O. Anderson, and J.E. Fox. 1991. *Health Psychology: Clinical Methods and Research,* ch. 7. New York: Macmillan: 159-196.

Youngston, R. M. 1993. *The Surgery Book: An Illustrated Guide to 73 of the Most Common Operations.* New York: St. Martin's Press.
This book presents exceptionally clear and detailed descriptions and tasteful illustrations of many common surgical procedures.

Chapter 1

Bennett, H.L., and E.A. Disbrow. 1993. "Preparing for Surgery and Medical Procedures." In *Mind-Body Medicine: How to Use Your Mind for Better Health,* edited by D. Goleman and J. Gurin. Yonkers, NY: Consumer Reports Books: 401-427.

Contrada, R.J., E.A. Leventhal, and J.R. Anderson. 1994. "Psychological Preparation for Surgery: Marshaling Individual and Social Resources to Optimize Self-Regulation." In *International Review of Health Psychology* 3, edited by S. Maes, H. Leventhal, and M. Johnston. New York: John Wiley & Sons, Ltd. 219-266.

Devine, E.C. 1992. "Effects of Psychoeducation Care for Adult Surgical Patients: A Meta-Analysis of 191 Studies." *Patient Education and Counseling* 19: 129-142.

Johnson, J.E., V.H. Rice, S.S. Fuller, and M.D. Endress. 1978. "Sensory Information, Instruction in a Coping Strategy, and Recovery from Surgery." *Research in Nursing and Health* 1(1): 4-17.

Johnston, M. 1988. "Impending Surgery." In *Handbook of Life Stress, Cognition and Health,* edited by S. Fisher and J. Reason. New York: John Wiley & Sons, Ltd. 79-100.

Johnston, M., and C. Vogele. 1993. "Benefits of Psychological Preparation for Surgery: A Meta-Analysis." *Annals of Behavioral Medicine* 15(4):245-256.

Kaloupek, D.G. 1987. "Recommendations for Psychological Intervention with Patients Undergoing Invasive Medical Procedures." *The Behavior Therapist* 10:33-39.

Kiecolt-Glaser, J.K., P.T. Marucha, W.B. Malarkey, A.M. Mercado, and R. Glaser. 1995. *Slowing of Wound Healing by Psychological Stress.* Lancet 346:1194-1196.

Linn, B.S., M.W. Linn, and N.G. Klimas. 1988. "Effects of Psychological Stress on Surgical Outcome." *Psychosomatic Medicine* 50:230-244.

Macho, J., and G. Cable. 1994. *Everyone's Guide to Outpatient Surgery*. Kansas City, MO: Sommerville House Books.

Matthews, A., and V. Ridgeway. 1981. "Personality and Surgical Recovery: A Review." *British Journal of Clinical Psychology* 2:243-260.

Miller, S.M. 1987. "Monitoring and Blunting: Validation of a Questionnaire to Assess Styles of Information-Seeking Under Threat." *Journal of Personality and Social Psychology* 52(2):345-353.

Sobel, D.S., and R. Ornstein. 1996. *The Healthy Mind, Healthy Body Handbook*. Los Altos, CA: Drx.

Youngson, Robert M. 1993. *The Surgery Book: An Illustrated Guide to 73 of the Most Common Operations*. New York: St. Martin's Press.

Chapter 2
General Information

American Psychiatric Association. 1994. *Diagnostic and Statistical Manual of Mental Disorders*, 4th ed. (DSM-IV). New York: Author.

Felton, B.J., T.A. Revenson, and G.A. Hinrichsen. 1984. "Stress and Coping in the Explanation of Psychological Adjustment Among Chronically Ill Adults." *Social Science and Medicine* 18:889-898.

Horne, D., P. Vatmanidis, and A. Careri. 1994. "Preparing Patients for Invasive Medical and Surgical Procedures I: Adding Behavioral and Cognitive Interventions." *Behavioral Medicine* 20:5-26.

Vitaliano, P.P., J. Russo, J.E. Carr, R.D. Maiuro, and J. Becker. 1985. "The Ways of Coping Checklist: Revision and Psychometric Properties." *Multivariate Behavioral Research* 20:3-26.

Volicer, B.J., and M.W. Bohannon. 1975. "A Hospital Stress Rating Scale." *Nursing Research* 24(5):352-359.

Volicer, B.J., M.A. Isenberg, and M.W. Burns. 1977. "Medical-Surgical Differences in Hospital Stress Factors." *Journal of Human Stress* 3:1-13.

Depression

Beck, A.T. 1979. *Cognitive Therapy and the Emotional Disorders*. New York: Meridian.

Burns, D.D. 1980. *Feeling Good: The New Mood Therapy*. New York: Avon Books.

Copeland, M.E. 1992. *The Depression Workbook*. Oakland, CA: New Harbinger Publications.

Padesky, C.A., and D. Greenberger. 1995. *Mind Over Mood*. New York: Guilford Press.

Anxiety

Barlow, D.H., and M. Craske. 1994. *Mastery of Your Anxiety and Panic*. Albany, NY: Graywind Publications.

Bourne, E.J. 1995. *The Anxiety and Phobia Workbook,* 2nd ed. Oakland, CA: New Harbinger Publications.

Zuercher-White, E. 1995. *An End to Panic: Breakthrough Techniques for Overcoming Panic Disorder.* Oakland, CA: New Harbinger Publications.

Anger

Novaco, R. 1975. *Anger Control: The Development and Evaluation of an Experimental Treatment.* Lexington, MA: D.C. Heath.

Potter-Efron, R., and P. Potter-Efron. 1995. *Letting Go of Anger.* Oakland, CA: New Harbinger Publications.

Williams, R., and V. Williams. 1993. *Anger Kills: Seventeen Strategies for Controlling the Hostility That Can Harm Your Health.* New York: Random House.

Chapter 3

AHCPR Practice Guidelines for Acute Pain Management: Operative or Medical Procedures and Trauma. 1992. Available free from the Agency for Health Care Policy and Research (AHCPR) Clearinghouse, P. O. Box 8547, Silver Springs, MD 20907, (800) 358-9295.

Anderson, L.A., and R.F. Dedrick. 1990. "Development of the Trust in Physician Scale: A Measure to Assess Interpersonal Trust in Patient-Physician Relationships." *Psychological Reports* 67:1091-1100.

Austin, E. 1995. "Are You at Risk?" *McCall's* (Nov.):88-90.

Autonomy Publishing Corporation, P.O. Box 1142, Dept. 172, Grand Central Station, New York, NY 10163, (800) 474-7416.
Publishes a book and audiotapes related to preparation for surgery.

Be Informed: Questions to Ask Your Doctor Before You Have Surgery. AHCPR Pub. No. 95-0027. Available from: Agency for Health Care Policy and Research (AHCPR) Publications Clearinghouse, P. O. Box 8547, Silver Springs, MD 20907, (800) 358-9295.

Leeds, D. 1992. *Smart Questions to Ask Your Doctor.* New York: HarperPaperbacks.

Ley, P. 1982. Studies of Recall in Medical Settings. *Human Learning* 1:223-233.

McCabe, J. 1994. *Surgery Electives: What to Know Before the Doctor Operates,* ch. 6. Santa Monica, CA: Carmania Books.

Roter, D.L. 1977. "Patient Participation in the Patient-Provider Interaction: The Effects of Patient Question-Asking on the Quality of Interaction, Satisfaction and Compliance." *Health Education Monographs* 5:281-315.

Chapter 4

AHCPR Practice Guidelines for Acute Pain Management: Operative or Medical Procedures and Trauma. 1992. Available free from the Agency for Health Care Policy and Research (AHCPR) Clearinghouse, P. O. Box 8547, Silver Springs, MD 20907, (800) 358-9295.

American Pain Society, 4700 W. Lake Avenue, Glenview, IL 60025-1485, (708) 375-4715. *Has many resources related to the study of pain.*

Bradley, E. 1994. *A Patient's Guide to Surgery.* Yonkers, NY: Consumer Reports Books.

Catalano, E.M. 1987. *The Chronic Pain Control Workbook.* Oakland, CA: New Harbinger Publications.

International Association for the Study of Pain, 909 NE 43rd Street., Suite 306, Seattle, WA 98105-6020, (206) 547-6409.

Kabat-Zinn, J. 1990. *Full Catastrophe Living: Using the Wisdom of Your Body and Mind to Face Stress, Pain, and Illness.* New York: Delacorte Press.

Liebeskind, J.C. 1991. "Pain *Can* Kill." *Pain* 44:3-4.

McCaffery, M., and A. Beebe. 1989. *Pain: Clinical Manual for Nursing Practice.* St. Louis, MO: C.V. Mosby.

Melzack, R., and P.D. Wall. 1982. *The Challenge of Pain.* New York: Basic Books.

Moyers, B. 1993. *Healing and the Mind.* New York: Doubleday.

Principles of Analgesic Use in the Treatment of Acute Pain and Cancer Pain, 3d ed. 1992. Committee Report for the American Pain Society, 4700 W. Lake Avenue, Glenview, IL 60025-1485, (708) 375-4715.

Ready, B.L., and W.T. Edwards, eds. 1992. *Management of Acute Pain: A Practical Guide.* Seattle, WA: International Association for the Study of Pain.

Rippa, C. 1992. Awareness: Wellspring (Summer). Christ Hospital and Medical Center, Oak Lawn, IL (708) 346-5064.

Sobel, D., and R. Ornstein. 1996. *The Healthy Mind, Healthy Body Handbook.* Los Altos, CA. Drx.

Woolf, C., and M. Chong. 1993. "Preemptive Analgesia—Treating Postoperative Pain by Preventing the Establishment of Central Sensitization." *Anesthesia, Analgesia* 77:362-379.

Chapters 5 and 6

Beck, A.T. 1979. *Cognitive Therapy and the Emotional Disorders.* New York: Meridian.

Bourne, E.J. 1995. *The Anxiety and Phobia Workbook,* 2d ed., ch. 9, 10. Oakland, CA: New Harbinger Publications.

Burns, D.D. 1980. *Feeling Good: The New Mood Therapy.* New York: Avon Books.

Davis, M., E.R. Eshelman, and M. McKay. 1995. *The Relaxation and Stress Reduction Workbook,* 4th ed. Oakland, CA: New Harbinger Publications.

Ellis, A. 1975. *A New Guide to Rational Living.* North Hollywood, CA: Wilshire Books.

McKay, M., M. Davis, and P. Fanning. 1981. *Thoughts and Feelings: The Art of Cognitive Stress Intervention.* Oakland, CA: New Harbinger Publications.

McKay, M., and P. Fanning. 1991. *Prisoners of Belief: Exposing and Changing Beliefs that Control Your Life.* Oakland, CA: New Harbinger Publications.

Sobel, D.S., and R. Ornstein. 1996. "Healthy Thinking." *Mental Medicine Update* 4(4):4-5.

Chapter 7

Benson, H. 1975. *The Relaxation Response*. New York: William Morrow.

Bourne, E.J. 1995. *The Anxiety and Phobia Workbook*, 2d ed. Oakland, CA: New Harbinger Publications, ch. 4.

Caudill, M.A. 1995. *Managing Pain Before It Manages You,.* ch. 3, 4. New York: Guilford.

Davis, M., E.R. Eshelman, and M. Mckay. 1995. *The Relaxation and Stress Reduction Workbook*, 4th ed. Oakland, CA: New Harbinger Publications.

Fried, Robert. 1993. "The Psychology and Physiology of Breathing." In *Behavioral Medicine, Clinical Psychology and Psychiatry*. New York: Plenum Press.

Furlong, M.W., and E. Essman. 1994. *Going Under: Preparing Yourself for Anesthesia*. New York: Autonomy Press.

Lehrer, P.M., and R.L. Woolfolk, eds. 1993. *Principles and Practice of Stress Management*, 2nd ed. New York: Guilford Press.

Sobel, D.S., and R. Ornstein. 1996. *The Healthy Mind, Healthy Body Handbook*, ch. 6. Los Altos, CA: Drx. Available from Drx, Box 176, Los Altos, CA 94023, (415) 948-6293.

Meditation

Benson, H. 1996. *Timeless Healing: The Power and Biology of Belief*. New York: Scribners.
Presents a biological model for the effects of belief. Highly recommended.

Goleman, D. 1988. *The Meditative Mind*. Los Angeles, CA: Tarcher.

Kabat-Zinn, J. 1993. "Mindfulness Meditation: Health Benefits of an Ancient Buddhist Practice." In *Mind/Body Medicine*, edited by D. Goleman and J. Gurin. Yonkers, NY: Consumer Reports Books.

Kabat-Zinn, J. 1990. *Full Catastrophe Living: Using the Wisdom of Your Body and Mind to Face Stress, Pain, and Illness*. New York: Delacort/Dell.
This book provides a detailed step-by-step instruction for mindfulness meditation for health and stress control.

Kabat-Zinn, J. 1994. *Wherever You Go There You Are: Mindfulness Meditation in Everyday Life*. New York: Hyperion. Presents essays and poems on mindfulness.

Kornfeld, J. 1993. *A Path With Heart: A Guide Through the Perils and Promises of a Spiritual Life*. New York: Bantam Books.

Levine, S.A. 1979. *A Gradual Awakening*. Garden City, NY: Anchor/Doubleday.

Mind/Body Institute, 101 Francis Street, Boston, MA 02215, (617) 632-9225.
Produces audio- and videotapes for relaxation and meditation practice.

Ram Dass. *Be Here Now*. 1971. New York: Crown.

Stress Reduction Clinic, University of Massachusetts, Medical Center, Worcester, MA 01655, (508) 856-1616. This program is directed by Dr. Jon Kabat-Zinn.

Stress Reduction Tapes, P. O. Box 547, Lexington, MA 02173. Tape 1: *Guided Body Scan/Mindfulness Yoga*; Tape 2: *Guided Sitting Meditation/Mindful Yoga*.
These tapes are used by Dr. Jon Kabat-Zinn at the UMMC Stress Reduction Clinic.

The World of Relaxation: A Video Program for Inpatient Education. Stress Reduction Video, University of Massachusetts Medical Center, 55 Lake Avenue, North, Worcester, MA 01655.
This video, produced by Dr. Jon Kabat-Zinn, is helpful in coping with the stress of health problems and hospitalization.

Taped Relaxation

Audio Prescriptives Foundation, Surgical Audiotape Series, 70 Maple Avenue, Katonah, NY 10536, (914) 232-6405. Contact Linda Rodgers.
These tapes contain originally composed anxiolytic music and relaxation instructions for use before, during, and after surgery, packaged in a manner that allows easy access in the hospital. We find these tapes to be exceptionally effective.

The Going Under, Preparing Yourself for Anesthesia Audio Cassettes. Autonomy Publishing Corp., P. O. Box 1142, New York, NY 10163.

New Harbinger Publications, Inc., 5674 Shattuck Avenue, Oakland, CA 94609, (800) 748-6273. Ask for the "Self-Help Catalog."

Intrinsic Developments, 410 E. Main Street, Mechanicsburg, PA 17055, (800) 354-2858. Surgical Preparation Tapes.
Included in their extensive selection of well-produced tapes for various problems, e.g., pain, headache, sleep and anxiety, are a series of three surgical preparation tapes designed to be used before, during, and after surgery. We have used these tapes extensively and our patients find them effective.

Chapter 8

Academy for Guided Imagery, P. O. Box 2070, Mill Valley, CA 94942. Relaxation and imagery books and tapes.

Achterberg, J. 1985. *Imagery in Healing: Shamanism and Modern Medicine.* Boston, MA: Shambhala Publications, Inc.

American Association of Therapeutic Humor, 222 S. Merrimac, Suite 303, St. Louis, MO 63105, (314) 863-6232.

Bourne, E.J. 1995. *The Anxiety and Phobia Workbook,* 2d ed. Oakland, CA: New Harbinger Publications.

Davis, M., E.R. Eshelman, and M. McKay. 1995. *The Relaxation and Stress Reduction Workbook,* 4th ed. Oakland, CA: New Harbinger Publications.

Fanning, P. 1988. *Visualization for Change.* Oakland, CA: New Harbinger Publications.

The Humor Project. 110 Spring Street, Saratoga Springs, NY 12866, (518) 587-8770. Publishes *Laughing Matters Magazine* and the *Humor Resources Catalogue.*

Klein, A. 1989. *The Healing Power of Humor.* Los Angeles, CA: Jeremy P. Tarcher.

Lusk, J.T. 1992. *30 Scripts for Relaxation Imagery and Inner Healing*, vol. 1, 2. Duluth, MN: Whole Person Associates.

McCaffery, M., and A. Beebe. 1989. *Pain: Clinical Manual for Nursing Practice*. St. Louis, MO: C.V. Mosby.

Sobel, D.S., and R. Ornstein. 1996. *The Healthy Mind, Healthy Body Handbook*, ch. 7. Los Altos, CA: Drx.

Whole Person Associates, Inc., 210 West Michigan, Duluth, MN 55802-1908, (213) 727-0500. Relaxation and imagery tapes and books.

Hypnosis

American Society of Clinical Hypnosis, 2200 East Devon Avenue, Suite 291, Des Plaines, IL 60018, (708) 297-3317.

Bennett, H.L., and E.A. Disbrow. 1993. "Preparing for Surgery and Other Medical Procedures." In *Mind/Body Medicine*, edited by D. Goleman and J. Gurin. Yonkers, NY: Consumer Reports Books.

Hadley, J., and C. Stuadacher. 1989. *Hypnosis for Change*. Oakland, CA: New Harbinger Publications.

Hilgard, E.R., and J.R. Hilgard. 1983. *Hypnosis in the Relief of Pain*. Los Altos, CA: William Kaufmann.

Orne, M.T., and D.F. Dinges. 1989. "Hypnosis." In *Comprehensive Textbook of Psychiatry*, 5th ed., edited by H.I. Kaplan and B.J. Sadock. Baltimore, MD: Williams and Wilkins.

Pratt, G.J., D.P. Wood, and B.M. Alman. 1984. *A Clinical Hypnosis Primer*. La Jolla, CA: Psychology and Consulting Associates Press.

Reeves, J.L., W.H. Redd, F.K. Storm, and R.Y. Minagawa. 1983. "Hypnosis in the Control of Pain During Hyperthermia Treatment of Cancer." In *Advances in Pain Research and Therapy* 5: 857-861, edited by J.J. Bonica, U. Lindblom, and A. Iggo. New York: Raven Press.

Spanos, N.P., and J.F. Chaves, eds. 1989. *Hypnosis: The Cognitive-Behavioral Perspective*. Buffalo, NY: Prometheus Press.

Spiegel, H., and D. Spiegel. 1978. *Trance and Treatment: Clinical Uses of Hypnosis*. New York: Basic Books.

Chapter 9

Bennett, H.L., and E.A. Disbrow. 1993. "Preparing for Surgery and Medical Procedures." In *Mind-Body Medicine: How to Use Your Mind for Better Health*, edited by D. Goleman and J. Gurin. Yonkers, NY: Consumer Reports Books: 401-427.

Eich, E., J. L. Reeves, and R. L. Katz. 1985. "Anesthesia, Amnesia, and the Memory/Awareness Distinction." *Anesthesia and Analgesia*. 64:1143–1148

Hado Music, Inc., 145 Hodencamp Road #204, Thousand Oaks, CA 91360, (805) 374-1923. Offers a selection of music for health.

Halpern, S. 1985. *Sound Health: The Music and Sounds That Make Us Whole*. San Francisco, CA: Harper & Row.

Maranto, C.D. 1993. "Music Therapy and Stress Management." In *Principles and Practice of Stress Management*, 2d ed., edited by P.M. Lehrer and R.L. Woolfolk. New York: Guilford Press.

New Harbinger Publications, Inc., 5674 Shattuck Avenue, Oakland, CA 94609, (800) 748-6273. Among other products, has audiotapes for visualization, relaxation, and anxiolytic music.

PIP Surgical Audiotape Series, Inc., 70 Maple Avenue, Katonah, NY 10536, (800) 588-5423. For information contact: Linda Rodgers, CSW.
Provides an audiotape series based on specific messages and anxiolytic music.

Rodgers, L. 1995. "Music for Surgery." *Advances: The Journal of Mind-Body Health* 11(3):49-57.

Whole Person Associates. 210 West Michigan, Duluth, MN 55802-1908, (800) 247-6789.
Offers a variety of audiotapes containing anxiolytic music, guided imagery, and relaxation exercises.

Chapter 10

Benor, D.J. 1990. "Survey of Spiritual Healing Research." *Complementary Medical Research* 4:9-33.

Benson, H. 1996. *Timeless Healing: The Power and Biology of Belief*. New York: Scribners.

Bourne, E.J. 1995. *The Anxiety and Phobia Workbook*, 2d ed., ch. 19. Oakland, CA: New Harbinger Publications.

Byrd, R.C. 1988. "Positive Therapeutic Effects of Intercessory Prayer in a Coronary Care Unit Population." *Southern Medical Journal* 81(7):826-829.

Dossey, L. 1993. *Healing Words: The Power of Prayer and the Practice of Medicine*. New York: HarperCollins.

Gallup, G.H., Jr. 1990. *Religion in America*. Princeton, NJ: Princeton Religion Research Center.

Kushner, H.S. 1981. *When Bad Things Happen to Good People*. New York: Avon Books.

Larson, D.B. 1993. *The Faith Factor: An Annotated Bibliography of Systematic Reviews and Clinical Research on Spiritual Subjects*, vol. 2. Boston, MA: John Templeton Foundation.

Levin, J.S. 1994. "Religion and Health: Is There an Association, Is It Valid, and Is It Causal?" *Social Science and Medicine* 38:1475-1482.

Levin, J.S., and P.L. Schiller. 1987. "Is There a Religious Factor in Health?" *Journal of Religion and Health* 26:9-36.

Matthews, D.A., D.B. Larson, and C.P. Barry. 1994. *The Faith Factor: An Annotated Bibliography of Clinical Research on Spiritual Subjects*, vol. 1. Boston, MA: John Templeton Foundation.

Orr, R.D., and G. Isaac. 1992. "Religious Variables Are Infrequently Reported in Clinical Research." *Family Medicine* 24:602-606.

Oxman, T.E., D.H. Freeman, Jr., and E.D. Manheimer. 1995. "Lack of Social Participation or Religious Strength and Comfort As Risk Factors for Death After Cardiac Surgery in the Elderly." *Psychosomatic Medicine* 57:5-15.

Pressman, P., J.S. Lyons, D.B. Larson, and J.J. Strain. 1990. "Religious Belief, Depression, and Ambulation Status in Elderly Women with Broken Hips." *American Journal of Psychiatry* 147:758-760.

Wallis, C. "Faith and Healing." *Time* (June 24, 1996):58-68.

Chapter 11

Bourne, E.J. 1995. *The Anxiety and Phobia Workbook*, 2d ed., ch. 4. Oakland, CA: New Harbinger Publications.

Culp, S. 1991. *Streamlining Your Life: A Five-Point Plan for Uncomplicated Living.* Cincinnati, OH: Writer's Digest Books.

Sobel, D.S., and R. Ornstein. 1996. *The Healthy Mind, Healthy Body Handbook*, ch. 14. Los Altos, CA: Drx.

Chapter 12

Alberti, R.E., and M. Emmons. 1974. *Your Perfect Right*, rev. ed. San Luis Obispo, CA: Impact Press.

Benson, H. 1996. *Timeless Healing: The Power and Biology of Belief.* New York: Scribners.

Bourne, E.J. 1995. *The Anxiety and Phobia Workbook*, 2d ed., ch. 14. Oakland, CA: New Harbinger Publications.

Bower, S.A., and G.H. Bower. 1991. *Asserting Yourself.* Reading, MA: Addison-Wesley Publishing.

Burns, D.D. 1989. *The Feeling Good Handbook.* New York: Penguin Books.

Caudill, M.A. 1995. *Managing Pain Before It Manages You,* ch. 8. New York: Guilford Press.

Davis, M., E.R. Eshelman, and M. McKay. 1995. *The Relaxation and Stress Reduction Workbook*, 4th ed. Oakland, CA: New Harbinger Publications.

Ferguson, T. 1993. "Working With Your Doctor." In *Mind-Body Medicine: How to Use Your Mind for Better Health*, edited by D. Goleman and J.Gurin. Yonkers, NY: Consumer Reports Books: 429-450.

Griffin, K. 1996. "They Should Have Washed Their Hands." *Health* (Nov.-Dec.): 82-90.

Kaplan, S.H., S.S. Greenfield, and J.E. Ware. 1989. "Assessing the Effects of Physician-Patient Interactions on the Outcomes of Chronic Disease." *Medical Care* 27(3):110-127.

McKay, M., M. Davis, and P. Fanning. 1983. *Messages: The Communication Book.* Oakland, CA: New Harbinger Publications.

Please forward questions and comments for Dr. Deardorff or Dr. Reeves to:

Preparing for Surgery
P. O. Box 18157
Beverly Hills, CA 90209

or you can contact us at our webpage at: www.surgeryprep.com.

Special Offer

Preparing for Surgery is available at discount prices when ordered in quantities of five or more copies. For details, call 1-800-748-6273 Monday-Friday from 9:00 AM to 5:00 PM Pacific Standard Time.

Other New Harbinger Self-Help Titles